CALIFORNIA STATE UNIVERSITY, SACRAMENTO

This book is due on the last date stamped below.
Failure to return books on the date due will result in assessment
of overdue fees.

World Health Organization
Geneva
1997

First edition, 1984
Second edition, 1997

WHO Library Cataloguing in Publication Data

Strategies for the prevention of blindness in national programmes : a primary health care
    approach. — 2nd ed.

   1.Blindness — prevention and control   2.Eye diseases — prevention and control
   3.Eye infections — prevention and control   4.National health programs   5.Primary health care

   ISBN 92 4 154492 9   (NLM Classification: WW 276)

TYPESET IN HONG KONG
PRINTED IN ENGLAND

95/10646—Best-set/Clays—7500

Contents

CONTENTS

Preface

This book was originally prepared by a working group for the WHO Programme for the Prevention of Blindness, and included contributions from several WHO Collaborating Centres. The book has been popular, enjoying a steady demand since its publication in 1984. When it sold out, it was decided to revise the book to include more recent developments, such as a simplified grading scheme for trachoma, the use of ivermectin against onchocerciasis and technological developments in cataract surgery. Furthermore, two chapters discussing childhood blindness and diabetic retinopathy have been added to the section "Methodological approaches to specific blinding conditions".

The WHO Programme for the Prevention of Blindness and Deafness gratefully acknowledges the valuable work done by past and present contributors. It is hoped that this book will continue to be widely used in planning and developing national programmes for the prevention of blindness.

B. Thylefors
Director
Programme for the Prevention of Blindness and Deafness
World Health Organization

1. Introduction and background

The concept of avoidable blindness

Blindness is a major health problem that has received relatively little attention in worldwide efforts to promote health. The vast majority of the world's blind live in developing countries, where infections, malnutrition and lack of eye care give rise to a high proportion of blindness, particularly in rural populations. Thus these countries have blindness rates that are 10–40 times greater than those of industrialized countries, where blindness is due mainly to degenerative and metabolic disorders related to ageing.

It has been estimated that there are at least 38 million blind people in the world, if blindness is defined as the inability to count fingers at a distance of 3 metres. This is the definition recommended by WHO (see Table 1). There are also an estimated 110 million people with low vision, i.e. visual acuity less than 0.3 (6/18).

A major portion of blindness in developing countries either can be cured, or could have been prevented, by a reasonable deployment of skills and resources. This is termed avoidable blindness. Blindness of infectious or nutritional origin can easily be prevented, and visual loss from cataract can be restored by simple surgery. Endemic trachoma and associated infections affect approximately 150 million people in the poorer rural communities of developing countries and can be controlled through hygienic measures such as face-washing, the application of antibiotic ointments in children and corrective lid surgery in adults. Malnutrition resulting in severe vitamin A deficiency can cause permanent blindness by damage to the cornea. This is particularly true in children living under conditions of general malnutrition who are affected by superimposed diseases such as measles, diarrhoea and acute respiratory infections that can aggravate their vitamin A status. Cataract, or opacity of the crystalline lens of the eye, occurs more frequently with advancing age and may affect more than 90% of those over 60 years of age worldwide. Cataract constitutes the major cause of easily curable blindness in most regions, as vision can be restored by simple and effective surgery. The parasitic infection

Table 1. Categories of visual impairment[a]

Category of visual impairment[b]	Visual acuity with best possible correction	
	Maximum less than:	Minimum equal to or better than:
1	6/18 3/10 (0.3) 20/70	6/60 1/10 (0.1) 20/200
2	6/60 1/10 (0.1) 20/200	3/60 1/20 (0.05) 20/400
3	3/60 1/20 (0.05) 20/400	1/60 (finger-counting at 1 metre) 1/50 (0.02) 5/300 (20/1200)
4	1/60 (finger-counting at 1 metre) 1/50 (0.02) 5/300 (20/1200)	Light perception
5	No light perception	
9	Undetermined or unspecified	

[a] Adapted from *International Statistical Classification of Diseases and Related Health Problems*, Tenth Revision. Geneva, World Health Organization, 1992.

[b] Categories of visual impairment 1 and 2 are referred to as "low vision", categories 3, 4 and 5 as "blindness", and category 9 as "unqualified visual loss". If the extent of the visual field is taken into account, patients with a field no greater than 10° but greater than 5° around central fixation should be placed in category 3 and patients with a field no greater than 5° around central fixation should be placed in category 4, even if visual acuity is not impaired.

onchocerciasis is a major cause of blindness in some African countries, and is also present in certain areas in Central and South America; control of onchocerciasis, which used to depend solely on control of its blackfly vector, can now also be achieved through the administration of ivermectin to target populations. Blindness due to ocular trauma, a fourth cause of avoidable blindness, can be controlled by preventive efforts at the community level and by early, appropriate treatment. A fifth cause is glaucoma, a group of diseases generally characterized by elevated internal pressure of the eye and resulting in visual impairment. It accounts for about 15% of all blindness. Its control depends on case-detection and treatment with eye drops or surgery.

The general lack of eye health services in underserved communities in developing countries is responsible for much blindness. Early treatment of infectious and nutritional eye disease is essential to prevent visual loss, and such treatment can often be delivered effectively by auxiliary health personnel. The simple guidelines for strategies of primary eye care presented in this publication should assist trained health workers in their efforts to deal effectively with most common eye diseases.

Blindness is a significant burden to society, in that the cost of lost productivity and of rehabilitation and education of the blind is very high and increasing. The swift and effective use of resources for the prevention of blindness will provide enormous savings in both money and human suffering. The cost of preventing blindness is only a small fraction of the expense of rehabilitation, so the cost-effectiveness of preventive measures, including surgery for cataract, is very high. The vast amount of human suffering attendant upon blindness, and the reduced quality of life it entails, can be gauged by the lower life expectancy of the blind in some developing countries.

Two principal objectives of the WHO Programme for the Prevention of Blindness and Deafness are to make essential eye care available to all populations and to eliminate avoidable blindness. Through effective programmes, national blindness rates can be reduced to less than 0.5%, with no more than 1% in individual communities. To achieve this, well-planned activities, originating at the national level, are required, using systematic community-based action to eliminate avoidable vision loss. At present, national plans for the prevention of blindness are being implemented or established in approximately 100 countries. However, unless rapid and systematic action is taken, the worldwide number of blind is likely to double by the year 2020.

Overview

This publication describes the essential components of a national blindness prevention programme that can be effectively integrated into an overall primary health care system. The methods that an individual country can use to implement a programme will necessarily depend on existing health care delivery and blindness prevention activities.

Many effective "vertical" blindness prevention activities, such as for trachoma or xerophthalmia control, have been broadened to include activities relevant to the prevention of other blinding conditions. In areas where there are no activities yet in place and a primary health care system is being developed, blindness prevention should be included as an integral component. Emphasis should be placed on developing activities at the primary (village) level, as they will benefit the greatest numbers. However, secondary and tertiary facilities should also be developed to provide continued training, stimulation and support to the rest of the system, and care for more complicated cases, and to raise gradually the level of sophistication and competence of the entire national programme.

Although effective interventions have been developed for some major blinding disorders, like trachoma, malnutrition, cataract and onchocerciasis, the methods of dealing with other problems such as glaucoma are still evolving. There is therefore a great need for applied research to improve the effectiveness of preventive measures.

General aspects of the primary health care approach to prevention of blindness

Primary health care consists of:

". . . essential health care based on practical, scientifically sound and socially acceptable methods and technology made universally accessible to individuals and families in the community through their full participation and at a cost that the community and country can afford to maintain at every stage of their development in the spirit of self-reliance and self-determination."[1]

The prevention of blindness should be an integral part of primary health care. There are three distinct, yet related, components in the primary health care approach, only the last of which requires direct interaction between a sick individual and medical personnel. They are:

— social and community developments that promote health through changes in behaviour and the environment and that lead to the reduction or elimination of factors contributing to ocular disease, e.g. the provision of adequate, safe water supplies, growing and consuming foods rich in provitamin A, construction and maintenance of pit-latrines;
— strengthening community cooperation to promote, within the family, the recognition and appropriate care of individuals at risk for blinding disease, such as adequate feeding and oral rehydration of children with severe measles or diarrhoea; immunization is also important (e.g. community awareness of eye care can be promoted by local committees);
— delivery of eye care to individuals with potentially blinding disorders (e.g. treatment and referral of infectious corneal ulcers by village-level workers or cataract surgery performed by mobile teams or at stationary facilities).

---

[1] *Primary health care. Report of the International Conference on Primary Health Care: Alma-Ata, USSR, 6–12 September 1978.* Geneva, World Health Organization, 1978 (Health For All Series, No. 1), p. 3.

Of the three components, community and social development may be the hardest to achieve, but will eventually have the greatest impact. In many areas of the world, blinding infections and malnutrition have practically disappeared following moderate socioeconomic advances, despite the absence of specific disease control activities. As social development activities require some alterations in entrenched practices, they are necessarily difficult to achieve and slow to produce a noticeable effect. Their long-term impact, however, will be considerable and will ultimately produce marked savings for health care systems.

The provision of curative services has the most obvious and immediate impact and has therefore long received a disproportionate share of attention and resources. None the less, disadvantaged communities throughout the world suffer from a lack of suitably trained personnel to treat existing disease. As it is possible as well as efficient to manage most eye diseases in the communities where they arise, emphasis should be placed on the development of primary eye care and a good referral system.

The development of eye health services

The prevention of blindness and the delivery of eye care should be integrated with general health services at all levels. Programmes should be based on available resources and technology that is appropriate for the country or region. The prevention of blindness requires a flexible approach and the incorporation of regular managerial and technical training for various categories of personnel. Programmes should be reviewed regularly, and improvements should be made that are consistent with economic growth and a social and cultural understanding of the population concerned.

Primary eye care

Primary eye care comprises a simple but comprehensive set of promotive, preventive and curative actions that can be carried out by suitably trained primary health workers, specialized auxiliary personnel or other interested people. The development and implementation of primary eye care activities will depend on the existing primary health care system. Locally available personnel and training programmes for primary health care can be used to promote and strengthen the delivery of eye care at the peripheral level. However, in areas without any existing primary health care system, services for primary eye care should be developed which could eventually evolve into more comprehensive health care activities.

The primary eye care worker should carry out promotive and preventive activities, focusing on education and community participation to prevent visual loss. The clinical activities involved in primary eye care consist of simple means of treating the three major eye symptoms presented by patients: inflamed ("red") eyes, loss of vision and pain in the eye. At the primary level, the health worker can manage these problems by definitive treatment, by referral after immediate treatment or by referral alone.

General guidelines for this have been developed (see section 4), but they must be adapted to the communities served.

Only a few medicines and other materials are necessary for primary eye care. At the very least, an antibiotic eye ointment (usually a tetracycline) is needed, but other drugs that may be useful are vitamin A capsules, a second antibiotic ointment and zinc sulfate drops (for mild irritations). Bandages, sticking plaster (tape) and eye shields are very useful for primary eye care workers, and optional equipment may include a simple chart to measure visual acuity and a hand torch.

The most important factor for primary eye care is the training of health workers to recognize eye conditions and to take appropriate action. Training manuals for primary health workers should therefore cover eye care. Primary eye care must, in turn, be supported by reinforcing training and by referral services at the secondary level.

Secondary eye care

Eye care facilities at the secondary level should provide for the definitive management of common blinding conditions such as cataract, trichiasis and entropion (inturned eyelids), ocular trauma, primary angle-closure glaucoma and corneal and intraocular infections. Secondary eye care activities are usually carried out in dispensaries or hospitals at the district or provincial level, by staff such as ophthalmic assistants, general practitioners trained in eye care or fully qualified ophthalmologists. This level of eye care should be integrated into the general medical infrastructure, making the fullest possible use of existing staff and equipment.

The secondary eye care centre plays an important role as the level to which patients who cannot be managed at the primary level are referred. Close liaison with the local health workers is therefore essential, and the staff at the secondary level should be actively involved in the training and supervision of local health personnel working in the field of eye care.

The management of less common blinding conditions, which may require sophisticated equipment and specialized staff, should normally not be carried out at the secondary level. Resources for treating such conditions (e.g. corneal grafting, retinal detachment surgery) are usually more efficiently provided in regional or national centres for tertiary eye care.

Tertiary eye care

Facilities for sophisticated eye care are often available in university hospitals or similar institutions. The eye care delivered at this level usually covers a variety of diagnostic and therapeutic services, but availability is often limited to urban populations. It is important for the staff of tertiary eye centres to be involved in training the various categories of health personnel in eye care, and for there to be managerial support for the work at the primary and secondary levels. Tertiary eye care units should also provide technical leadership and play a leading role in the promotion of public health ophthalmology, including research related to the delivery of eye care. Support should also be given for the regular restocking of ophthalmic drugs and supplies at the primary and secondary levels, and in the assessment of locally prevalent disorders, e.g. trachoma.

Mobile eye services

Mobile ophthalmic teams may fulfil the function of delivering primary and secondary eye care in areas where such services are lacking. These units may also give valuable support to existing eye care services, particularly in the epidemiological and clinical assessment of specific blinding disorders. Mobile "eye camps" have been successfully used in certain countries to provide cataract surgery and refractive services, e.g. spectacles, at the peripheral level. These surgical teams can also perform optical iridectomies, a simple procedure that can restore useful vision to some individuals with central corneal opacities.

Mobile eye services may be relied upon for efficient intervention against blinding diseases in certain areas. However, it is important to ensure the continuity and follow-up of activities initiated by such teams, and to have close collaboration with the local health personnel and the communities concerned, e.g. by initiating health education activities. These services should be of a temporary nature and should eventually be replaced by a suitably located permanent infrastructure for eye health care.

2. National programmes[1] for the prevention of blindness

---

[1] The term "national programme", used throughout this book, implies a range of coordinated activities, based on a national policy and plan but implemented by means of the general health services system.

Basic concepts

National programmes for the prevention of blindness need central organization to determine priorities, mobilize and allocate resources, provide support at all levels of eye care, organize training and health education, and monitor and evaluate programme activities. Blindness prevention programmes may either evolve from programmes designed to control specific diseases (e.g. trachoma) or be established because excessive rates of blindness have been recognized.

National programmes should be based on the human and financial resources actually, as well as potentially, available to meet the goals set. Blindness prevention should be firmly based on primary health care, but it also requires the provision of definitive secondary care, especially the treatment of acute blinding conditions (e.g. corneal ulcers) and the surgical cure of cataract. Government policies should foster not only the training of ophthalmic personnel, but also their retention and equitable geographical distribution in the country and the fullest possible utilization of their resources.

The delivery of essential eye health services at the peripheral level should be an integral component of primary health care, and should include the promotion of eye health as well as the prevention and treatment of blinding conditions.

National programmes should organize and coordinate activities at all levels. These activities should include the following:

— assessment surveys to identify communities with a high prevalence of avoidable blindness and to determine the causes of such blindness;
— formulation of objectives and development of intervention strategies;
— training of personnel to take effective roles at all levels of the programme;
— development and provision of support for primary eye care;
— promotion and organization of individual and community participation in blindness prevention activities through health education;

— maintenance and monitoring of activities at all levels to ensure that they fit the needs of the programme;
— organization of special interventions to reduce excessive blindness caused by specific problems;
— evaluation of the impact of the programme.

Planning

National programmes should allow the greatest possible initiative and innovation by health workers at all levels, particularly in primary eye care. In some instances, independently organized and administered units (e.g. charitable eye hospitals) can offer vital services and should be encouraged if they contribute to the goals of blindness prevention.

Those features of a national programme that should be organized and administered at the national level (or provincial level in large countries) include the following:

- Establishment of a national committee or other authority to promote, initiate and coordinate blindness prevention policy development.
- Statement of a national policy for the prevention of blindness.
- Establishment of an office of national coordination for operational planning, monitoring and evaluation.
- Identification of personnel, facilities and programmes already active in the prevention of blindness.
- Assessment of blindness and blinding conditions through:
  — collection and review of existing information;
  — assessment surveys.
- Formulation of a plan of action and strategies with the identification and analysis of required tasks.
- Implementation of a primary eye care approach.
- Strengthening of secondary and tertiary facilities to support primary eye care.
- Temporary utilization of mobile units (when applicable) and organization of other outreach activities.
- Medical management and prevention of the major blinding disorders.
- Training and continuing education of personnel:
  — primary health care workers;
  — specialized ophthalmic auxiliary staff;

- — general physicians;
- — ophthalmologists.
- Supervision, motivation and evaluation of personnel at all levels, and provision of suitable career structures.
- Promotion of health education and community participation.
- Provision of:
  - — salary and necessary expenses for personnel;
  - — equipment, supplies and transport.
- Promotion of local industries and appropriate technology, e.g. low-cost spectacles, local preparation of eye drops or basic diagnostic equipment.
- Mobilization of financial and other resources:
  - — from national government, private funds or donations;
  - — from governmental agencies;
  - — from nongovernmental organizations;
  - — from intergovernmental agencies.
- Development of a comprehensive management information system.
- Evaluation:
  - — measurement of the time, cost and performance of programme activities;
  - — measurement of the effect on blindness rates and the prevalence of specific disorders;
  - — assessment of other useful indicators, such as the development of eye health services, community participation and changes in social and economic factors related to visual disability and its prevention.

Mobilization of resources

National resources

National programmes can make use of health services that are already carrying out eye care in the country. The identification of both governmental and nongovernmental resources is an important initial step in programme development and, together with an assessment of current needs, is critical for mobilizing resources.

With an inventory of existing activities and a carefully prepared plan of action, a strong case can be made for increasing the resources available for the prevention of blindness. External resources and assistance may more easily be obtained after a firm national commitment has been established. The specific ways in which this external support would strengthen the programme should be described in detail.

It is necessary to increase public awareness of blindness and its prevention in order to establish consensus on the need for a national blindness prevention programme. This can in part be generated by the support of influential individual "opinion-makers" or celebrities, professional societies and the print, television and other media. If a favourable climate of opinion has been created, the government will find it easier to allocate additional resources.

Nongovernmental sources and voluntary agencies may already be making a substantial contribution to blindness prevention through subsidized hospitals and clinics. Although these voluntary efforts do not have to be modified, their contribution to the national plan should be recognized. Every effort should be made to obtain support from the nongovernmental sector, whether in the form of financial contributions, volunteer personnel or donations of supplies, materials and facilities. The long-term sustainability of these programmes should be promoted and encouraged.

International cooperation

Through its Programme for the Prevention of Blindness and Deafness WHO can, upon request, offer assistance to national programmes in the organizing phase as well as in specific aspects of blindness prevention. Other organizations and bodies of the United Nations system, such as the United Nations Children's Fund (UNICEF), the United Nations Development Programme (UNDP) and the World Bank, can also make valuable contributions to the development process that will ultimately reduce the level of avoidable blindness.

A number of international nongovernmental organizations are active in blindness prevention, and these may be able to supply temporary technical staff and provide supplies, equipment and training opportunities.

Bilateral programmes between governments usually involve the transfer of financial resources. Such arrangements can create a greater sense of responsibility between the countries involved and act as a source of support for a prevention of blindness programme.

Technical cooperation between developing countries can provide another mechanism to support the prevention of blindness. Regional and subregional collaboration should be encouraged in specific fields, such as training of personnel and organization of disease control programmes.

Initiation of national programmes for the prevention of blindness

Once a national plan for the prevention of blindness has been formulated, steps should be taken to ensure its rapid implementation. During the early phase, the programme will have to rely on resources available within the country, which makes it essential that resources be utilized optimally.

The following measures should be considered in the initial phase of programme implementation. The medical and administrative staff who will manage the programme at the central as well as the peripheral level should be appointed and briefed about their new responsibilities. It is of particular importance to identify responsible health administrators at the provincial, district and community levels, in accordance with existing administrative divisions. After having received appropriate information and training, the medical administrators should identify resources for blindness prevention within the existing local infrastructure and ensure the integration of new activities with existing ones. Short national workshops or seminars for the local medical officers and administrators who will be involved in the management of blindness prevention have proved to be a useful and efficient means of imparting the necessary information and training.

The development of a management information system for eye care should be included as an integral part of the national health information system. Such a system should collect, analyse and disseminate the data required for planning, management, monitoring and evaluation.

The training of auxiliary health personnel in eye care should begin in the initial phase of a blindness prevention programme, even where the availability of equipment or teaching staff is limited. Valuable experience can be gained in trial courses for a few pupils, which will considerably facilitate the planning and allocation of resources for training on a large scale. Training activities for personnel at the primary and intermediate levels will have been elaborated in the planning phase of the programme and can be implemented on a wider scale when appropriate. A detailed inventory of available training facilities at various levels should be made and utilized accordingly. The future personnel requirements (i.e. teaching staff), as well as the need for training aids, documentation and teaching equipment, should be clearly identified and listed to facilitate the mobilization of appropriate resources. It is of particular importance to begin training village health workers at an early stage, in order to ensure the participation and involvement of local communities in the national programme.

A detailed inventory of dispensaries, health centres, eye clinics and other institutions for the delivery of eye care at the primary, secondary and tertiary levels should be made. The existing infrastructure for eye care should accordingly be clearly defined for each local administrative division. The personnel, equipment and supplies needed to strengthen this network and to establish an adequate referral system should be analysed and compiled in a form suitable for funding requests.

A reliable system for the supply of drugs and other ophthalmic supplies should be worked out for each level of eye care delivery. This system can often be integrated into the general medical supply system, but particular attention must be paid to remote rural areas, where the shortage of health personnel may necessitate special supply measures. The inventory of ophthalmic supplies should be periodically checked by supervisory staff in order to track consumption.

The participation of the community should be ensured from the initial stages by encouraging people's acceptance of the programme. The potential risks of certain indigenous health practices and taboos may need to be highlighted and gradually overcome by sustained health education.

3. Primary eye care

Definitions of primary eye care

Primary eye care is a vital component of primary health care and includes the promotion of eye health and the prevention and treatment of conditions that may lead to visual loss.

Primary eye care implies the first provision of promotive, preventive and therapeutic measures for eye health to an individual or a community. Such measures may be provided at different levels of sophistication, depending on local conditions and resources. However, primary eye care should also be an integral part of primary health care, in view of the existing situation in most developing countries, where avoidable blindness constitutes a major public health problem. In this context, priority should be given to identification of the essential eye care that should be delivered at the most peripheral level. The implementation of primary eye care should also be adapted as far as possible to locally available personnel and existing training programmes. In areas without a primary health care system, primary eye care services should be developed and can eventually evolve into a primary health care system.

Primary eye care needs to be supported and sustained by an adequate referral system. This implies conducting regular short training courses for, and the participation of, primary health workers in activities such as those of mobile surgical teams.

Primary eye care activities

Promotive and preventive activities

In order to promote eye health and prevent the loss of sight, the primary health care worker should disseminate information to as many people as possible in the community. The information should include the location where treatment is available and encourage patients to seek out and comply with treatment and report for follow-up care as advised. Much of this information can be imparted to specific target groups such as village leaders, community councils, administrative authorities, schoolteachers and pupils, as well as to individual households and patients.

The primary health care worker must be an effective educator, capable of making the community aware that the majority of blinding diseases are either preventable or curable. He or she should also instruct people in personal and environmental hygiene, nutrition, sanitation and protection of the eye.

The primary health care worker should stimulate individual and community participation in activities to prevent blindness, and become actively involved in community-based treatment programmes, for example against trachoma and xerophthalmia. He or she should also alert the local community to, and should follow up on, activities initiated by higher-level eye care services or mobile units. Such activities may include the supervision of treatment schemes and the reassessment of results of eye services delivered at other levels, e.g. results of trichiasis operations.

Clinical activities

With regard to clinical activities, a distinction should be made between conditions that ought to be:

— recognized and treated by the primary health care worker;
— recognized and referred after treatment has been initiated;
— recognized and referred for treatment.

Conditions to be recognized and treated by a trained primary health care worker

Conjunctivitis and lid infections

Acute conjunctivitis is recognized by redness of the globe and palpebral conjunctiva and a purulent discharge without any loss of vision. This should be treated with frequent applications of antibiotic drops or ointment by the patient or a family member. If there is no improvement in 3 days, the patient should be referred.

Ophthalmia neonatorum—a red eye with lid swelling and discharge— occurs in infants in the first few days after birth and is often caused by a maternal gonococcal infection. Conjunctivitis in the newborn is a serious and potentially blinding disorder that requires immediate and intensive topical and systemic antibiotic treatment, ideally at the secondary- or tertiary-level hospital.

Treatment should be carried out immediately with topical tetracycline 1% ointment 4–6 times daily in conjunction with systemic antibiotic treatment. It may be necessary to continue treatment for 2 weeks or longer until the conjunctivitis disappears. The eyes should be cleansed frequently to keep them free of discharge.

To prevent ophthalmia neonatorum, all newborn infants should be treated immediately after delivery with a single application of tetracycline 1% eye ointment or with silver nitrate 1% drops in both eyes (Crede's prophylaxis), following cleansing of the closed eyelids. Birth attendants and midwives should be instructed in how to apply this prophylaxis to the eyes of every newborn infant.

Trachoma is a chronic, endemic conjunctivitis often associated with seasonal epidemics of purulent conjunctivitis. If it is endemic, areas in which mass treatment is required should be determined. The treatment consists of the application twice daily of tetracycline 1% ointment to all children for 5 consecutive days each month for 6 months each year. Primary health workers should participate in these treatments and learn to recognize active trachoma and the resultant inturned eyelashes and eyelids (trichiasis and entropion). Further recommendations for trachoma control are given in section 4.

Allergic conjunctivitis and *irritative conjunctivitis* include most of the minor conditions producing chronic redness and itching without discharge or visual loss, such as blepharitis (lid margin infection), allergic conditions and irritation from dust. These conditions are treated with zinc sulfate drops for short periods. Corticosteroid preparations should never be used in field conditions by auxiliary personnel or without proper supervision for the treatment of conjunctivitis or other eye inflammation.

Lid lesions include styes (acute abscesses) and chalazia (chronic fatty cysts). These should be treated by the application of warm compresses or other means of warming the eye and by the application of antibiotic ointment for 3 days. Chalazia may require surgical treatment and therefore referral to secondary-level hospitals or mobile services.

Trauma

Subconjunctival haemorrhages appear suddenly as bright red patches on the white of the eye without discharge, visual loss or pain. The condition does not require treatment, but the patient should be reassured that it is not serious and heals rapidly. Subconjunctival haemorrhages associated with pain or visual loss should be referred.

Conjunctival foreign bodies under the eyelids, especially the upper eyelid, should be investigated by proper eversion of the lids. They can be removed with twisted cotton wool or a clean piece of cloth, following which antibiotic ointment should be applied.

Corneal foreign bodies usually produce redness, pain and tearing. They may be detected by the naked eye, but a magnifying glass or loupe is useful to identify and localize them. They may also be detected by irregularities in the surface reflection of a window or door on the cornea. Gentle scraping with a small blunt instrument, a folded piece of paper or a cotton-tipped applicator may remove superficial corneal foreign bodies. After removal, antibiotic ointment should be applied. If the foreign body cannot be removed easily, the patient should be referred to the secondary level.

Corneal abrasions are due to the loss of the superficial layer of cells on the surface of the cornea, usually following a minor injury to the eye, e.g. a fingernail scratch. They can be detected by the presence of an irregular surface reflection on an otherwise clear cornea and are treated by the application of antibiotic ointment and of a sterile eye patch, if available. The antibiotic application is repeated daily as long as the eye is painful.

Ecchymosis of the lids ("black" or bruised eyelids) does not need treatment if the vision has not been affected.

Hyphaema, blood behind the cornea, has the appearance of a dark red stain of the cornea (often with a fluid level) that may hide the pupil and iris. Patients with hyphaema usually have some visual loss. They should rest for 5 days. They must *not* be given aspirin or any other salicylic acid derivatives. If there is severe pain or nausea and vomiting, or if the blood does not disappear, at least in part, within 5 days, the patient should be referred to an ophthalmic centre.

Vitamin A deficiency

Potentially blinding vitamin A deficiency (xerophthalmia and keratoma-lacia) usually occurs in children under 6 years of age with malnutrition. It can be manifested as:

— night blindness (for instance, a child who cannot see or find its mother in a darkened room);
— foamy spots on the white of the eyeball on either side of the cornea (Bitot's spots);
— dry eye, in which the cornea appears to be roughened and dull and does not have a moist appearance (xerophthalmia);
— corneal ulcers, which may occur in a severely malnourished child, particularly after measles. In such a case, although the child may not complain of pain, a black spot may appear on the surface of the cornea where the iris has pushed through.

These cases should all be treated with 110 mg (200 000 IU) of retinyl palmitate (vitamin A) orally for 2 successive days. All children with corneal ulcers should receive vitamin A whether or not a deficiency is suspected (and be referred as indicated below). Further recommendations for the control of blinding malnutrition are given in section 4.

Conditions to be recognized and referred after treatment has been initiated

It is assumed that secondary- or tertiary-level centres are available for referral. However, in some areas, access to such centres may be limited, difficult or delayed; under such circumstances, the initial treatment given should be continued.

Corneal ulcers

Corneal ulcers can be recognized as red, painful eyes, usually with some decreased vision; they frequently cause blindness of the affected eye. The surface reflection of the cornea is irregular and there is often a white spot. These potentially blinding conditions require urgent and expert attention. It is important that the primary health care worker recognize the condition and initiate treatment by cleansing and by application of a topical antibiotic. The patient should be referred immediately to a secondary-level centre.

Lacerations or perforating injuries of the eyeball

Lacerations and perforations are caused by trauma to the eye. The eye is usually red and painful, with visual loss. There is often a black spot protruding through the wound (the iris or uvea). The eye should be protected with a shield, and systemic antibiotic treatment administered if available. Eye ointment should be avoided. The patient should be referred urgently for further action.

Lid lacerations

Patients with large lid lacerations and those with lacerations involving the lid margin should be referred, after initial gentle cleansing and padding of the injury. Systemic antibiotics may be administered, if available, before referral.

Entropion and trichiasis

Inturned eyelids (entropion) or eyelashes rubbing on the cornea (trichiasis) are most common in association with blinding trachoma, but may occur for other reasons. The patient usually complains of a scratching sensation on the eye. The inturned eyelashes can be detected with a good light directed at the lid margin, and the lids slightly rolled away from the eye while the patient looks up and then down.

Such patients should have eyelid surgery as soon as it is convenient. If the locality is visited regularly by a trachoma surgery team, a list of potential patients should be kept for the team. Otherwise, patients should be referred to the nearest eye service for surgery. As a temporary measure to prevent damage to the cornea and relieve symptoms, the inturned eyelashes can be pulled out with epilation forceps, and antibiotic ointment applied at least once daily until surgery can be performed.

Burns

Chemical burns should be treated by prolonged, immediate irrigation with water, with the eyelids held wide open. Antibiotic ointment, if available, should be applied before referral.

Thermal burns should be treated by application of antibiotic ointment, and the patient referred if there is serious skin damage.

Conditions that should be recognized and referred for treatment

Painful red eye with visual loss

Patients who present with painful red eyes and visual loss should be referred immediately.

Cataract

Cataract is an opacity of the lens of the eye. Patients with cataract have a gradual loss of vision not accompanied by pain. In advanced cases, the pupil appears to be chalky-white or greenish-grey in colour. These patients should be referred as soon as convenient to the nearest eye service for surgery. Further recommendations for the management of cataract are given in section 4.

Pterygium

Pterygium is a red, fleshy growth on the surface of the eye that grows over the surface of the cornea and may eventually impair vision. If the vision is affected, the patient should be referred to the nearest eye service as soon as convenient.

Visual loss

Patients whose vision has decreased and is worse than 0.3 (6/18) in either eye should be referred.

Personnel and training

Minimum qualifications for selection

Primary health care workers should be responsible for the delivery of primary eye care, and this should be an integral component of their duties. In order to perform these tasks effectively, candidates must be able to read and write. For efficiency, it is preferable to have workers who are selected by, or at least acceptable to, the community.

Training

Training should be simple, practical and task-oriented. It should be carried out, as far as possible, in or close to the community to be served and should preferably be directed by the supervisor, who would also be responsible for evaluation. Wherever feasible, existing health facilities can be utilized for group training.

Supervision

The primary health care worker should be supervised through regular visits of secondary-level personnel, e.g. an ophthalmologist, ophthalmic medical assistant, general physician or other competent health practitioner.

Records and reporting

Records should preferably be kept in a notebook indicating the following details: name, age, sex, locality, complaint or symptoms, provisional diagnosis and treatment given.

The primary health care worker should report to the supervisor during his or her routine visits through the presentation of relevant information from the record book.

Refresher courses

Refresher courses should be provided periodically by the supervisor or other suitable personnel, either at the community level or, if possible, at a training centre.

Evaluation of training

Evaluation of the training and the performance of the primary health care worker should be carried out by the supervisor, by utilizing the record book and personally assessing the fieldwork. An overall evaluation of the prevalence of the blinding conditions in the community and the effectiveness of the role played by the primary health care worker should be the responsibility of suitably qualified personnel.

Supplies and equipment for primary eye care

Local conditions should guide the choice of drugs and equipment from these lists. To avoid the loss of or shortfalls in supplies and drugs, it is recommended that there be regular inspection and auditing.

Drugs

Basic drug supplies for primary eye care consist of:

— tetracycline 1% eye ointment;
— chloramphenicol or other antimicrobial preparation for topical use in the eye;
— zinc sulfate 0.2% eye drops;
— vitamin A capsules—110 mg retinyl palmitate (200 000 IU);
— silver nitrate 1% eye drops—an alternative to tetracycline for use in the newborn as a prophylactic for ophthalmia neonatorum.

Eye drops and ointments containing pilocarpine, atropine or corticosteroids should not be provided at the primary level.

It is desirable for the supply of ophthalmic drugs to primary health care centres to be standardized and uniform, in order to enhance availability and reduce costs.

Supplies and equipment

Most communities will find the following supplies indispensable:

— optotypes—these should be adapted to local needs and could include Landolt ring, Snellen chart, E types or Sjögren's hand chart, either as single optotypes or as a simplified multiple optotype chart;
— electric torch and batteries;

— hand magnifying lens;
— epilation forceps (in trachoma-endemic areas);
— dressings—eye pads, bandages, sticking plaster, eye shields.

Wherever feasible, the local production of items such as bandages, shields and epilation forceps should be encouraged.

Training material

The training of a primary health care worker in the field of eye care will require teaching material such as manuals, recognition cards and posters. Such material should be simple, durable and obtainable at a relatively low cost.

Primary eye care is an essential part of primary health care, and the importance of promoting eye health at the community level should be stressed. Training material for primary health care workers in blindness prevention should include promotional material designed to encourage community participation.

Training material on the following subjects could be included:

- *Methods of examination* (to be illustrated by diagrams or photographs)
  - — taking and assessing the patient's history;
  - — assessment and recording of visual acuity;
  - — inspection of the eye and the lids;
  - — exposure of the conjunctiva of the lower lid;
  - — eversion of the conjunctiva of the upper lid;
  - — inspection of the globe in different directions of gaze;
  - — examination of the eyes of infants.
- *Clinical conditions.* The manual should outline the conditions to be recognized and treated by the primary health care worker and those needing referral, as listed in section 3. Suitable illustrations, with brief and clear descriptions, should be used.
- *Methods of treatment*
  - — cleansing and irrigating the eye;
  - — applying eye drops and ointment;
  - — application of eye pads and shields, and strapping and bandaging.

4. Methodological approaches to specific blinding conditions

Introduction

The basic features of the major blinding diseases and conditions in developing countries, and the means of controlling them, are discussed in the following pages. Please refer to "References and selected further reading", p. 102, for references to more detailed discussions of individual diseases. A particularly useful aid is the WHO eye examination record,[1] which describes in detail practical techniques for assessment of blindness and blinding conditions through surveys.

---

[1] *WHO eye examination record* (unpublished document WHO/PBL/EER III/1988; available on request from Programme for the Prevention of Blindness and Deafness, World Health Organization, 1211 Geneva 27, Switzerland).

Trachoma

Present state of knowledge

Endemic trachoma is still a major cause of blindness in rural communities of the developing world. Trachoma and associated infections are estimated to affect approximately 150 million people, most of them in the poorer rural communities of the developing world, especially in arid areas. There are probably some 6 million people who have been rendered blind or severely visually disabled by trachoma, and a much larger number have suffered some loss of vision. Trachoma can be controlled, and blindness and visual loss prevented, by relatively simple and inexpensive measures.

Description

Trachoma is a chronic inflammation of the eye leading to red, thickened membranes covering the inside of the eyelid and opacity of the cornea. The causative agent of trachoma is *Chlamydia trachomatis*, but infections with other bacteria and with viruses often contribute to the disease process.

Milder degrees of trachomatous inflammation may undergo spontaneous resolution. While trachoma may heal with no permanent damage, severe forms lead to blinding damage to the cornea. Frequent, repeated episodes of disease produce conjunctival scarring which can cause inward deviation of eyelashes (trichiasis) or of the lid margin (entropion). The abrasion of the cornea by wiry lashes, and defects in lid closure, frequently result in corneal ulceration, followed by scarring and visual loss. The final visual acuity may range from normal vision to total blindness. It is possible, then, to distinguish individuals and communities with blinding trachoma from those with non-blinding trachoma.

Persons with either condition may have signs of conjunctival inflammation, indicating active trachoma (presumably infectious), or scarring of the conjunctiva or other signs without inflammation, indicating inactive or healed trachoma.

Etiology

Infections of the eye with *C. trachomatis* occur in two distinct epidemiological situations. The first is the potentially blinding disease of developing countries that is spread by eye-to-eye transmission of infection and is best defined as endemic trachoma. It is almost invariably caused by serotype A, B or C of *C. trachomatis.*

Infection of the eye by the sexually transmitted *C. trachomatis* (serotype D, E, F, G, H, I, J or K) produces an eye disease that is often indistinguishable from the inflammatory phase of endemic trachoma. Milder cases are usually called "inclusion conjunctivitis", but the term "paratrachoma" conveniently applies to the whole spectrum of disease resulting from eye infections with sexually transmitted chlamydiae. Infection of newborns by sexually transmitted strains of *C. trachomatis* can cause conjunctivitis, pneumonia and gastrointestinal infection. Sporadic eye infections with sexually transmitted *C. trachomatis* strains (serotypes D–K) rarely produce permanent visual loss, but chlamydial respiratory tract infections in infants and genital tract infections in adults are important health problems in most populations.

Some communities with potentially blinding trachoma also have annual or biennial epidemics of non-chlamydial conjunctivitis clearly associated with increased numbers of eye-seeking flies. In other communities, trachoma is often associated with a constant level of bacterial and viral conjunctivitis throughout the year. The combination of non-chlamydial conjunctivitis and repeated episodes of active trachoma increases the severity of disease, producing more conjunctival scarring and blinding complications. Long-term follow-up studies have shown that the severity of trachomatous conjunctivitis in childhood is directly related to potentially blinding trichiasis and entropion in adult life.

Epidemiology

Trachoma has a worldwide distribution. At present, blinding trachoma is a major public health problem in parts of Africa, the Eastern Mediterranean region, the drier regions of the Indian subcontinent, South-East Asia and elsewhere in the Western Pacific region and parts of Oceania. Pockets of blinding trachoma also exist in Central and South America, the Caribbean and Australia. Non-blinding trachoma is present in these same areas, as well as in a much broader region that includes many of the drier subtropical and tropical countries.

In eastern Asia, Europe and North America, trachoma regressed and disappeared with the rising living standards that accompanied industrialization and economic development. Thus, under the living conditions prevailing in developed countries and in better-off urban communities of developing countries, trachoma is rarely transmitted and, if contracted, is mild.

In the most heavily affected communities, most children are infected by the age of 1 or 2 years with peak rates of active trachoma from 2 to 7 years. By adolescence the prevalence of active disease starts to decline, but some adults continue to have episodes of active disease. Because children constitute such a large proportion of the population in areas with endemic trachoma, children with active disease are the chief source of trachomatous infection in the community.

Severe conjunctival scarring is the outcome of moderate to severe inflammatory disease in childhood. These scars slowly contract, causing the lashes to abrade the cornea. Corneal lesions from this constant trauma appear more frequently after the age of 40 years. In countries where infectious childhood trachoma has disappeared, there may still be a large number of people requiring corrective lid surgery for trichiasis and entropion to prevent late corneal scarring.

It has long been known that trachoma is associated with poverty and that, with economic development, the active disease disappears or its severity and prevalence decrease. Among the environmental and behavioural features of greatest importance are the presence of young children in the household, the failure to wash young children daily, crowding and the unavailability of latrines or safe water. In addition, inadequate disposal of human and animal wastes leads to large fly populations, with frequent reinfection of children's eyes with chlamydial and other microbial organisms. It is the subsequent repeated episodes of active trachoma that cause progressive conjunctival scarring.

Diagnosis

The upper tarsal conjunctiva has been selected as a convenient index of trachomatous inflammation in the eye as a whole. A simple grading system of the key signs of trachoma has been developed for the assessment of trachoma and its complications by general health workers. These key signs are the following:

- *Trachomatous inflammation, follicular (TF)*: The presence of five or more follicles in the upper tarsal conjunctiva. Follicles are small, elevated, avascular lesions (at least 0.5 mm in diameter) involving the inner, conjunctival surface of the upper lid.
- *Trachomatous inflammation, intense (TI)*: Pronounced inflammatory thickening of the tarsal conjunctiva that obscures more than half of the normal deep tarsal vessels. The tarsal conjunctiva appears red, rough and thickened.

- *Trachomatous scarring (TS)*: The presence of scarring in the tarsal conjunctiva. Scars are easily visible as white lines, bands or sheets in the tarsal conjunctiva.
- *Trachomatous trichiasis (TT)*: At least one eyelash rubs on the eyeball. Evidence of recent removal of inturned eyelashes should also be graded as trichiasis.
- *Corneal opacity (CO)*: Easily visible corneal opacity over the pupil. The pupil margin is blurred viewed through the opacity.

A fuller grading system of the clinical signs of trachoma is available[1] which provides a detailed description of these and other signs for research purposes and for use by ophthalmologists and other specially trained personnel.

A community with blinding trachoma can be recognized by the presence of people with severe visual loss due to corneal opacity and a substantial prevalence of potentially disabling trachomatous lesions, particularly trichiasis and entropion. These irreversible changes appear as the long-term outcome of prolonged or recurrent inflammatory disease of moderate or severe intensity. Communities with non-blinding trachoma have a low prevalence of potentially blinding lesions and do not have a substantial prevalence of visual loss due to trachoma. However, in communities where economic development has occurred, although infectious trachoma may have disappeared a substantial proportion of adults may still manifest potentially blinding trachomatous lesions.

In communities with active trachoma, chlamydial infection is always present, but other ocular microbial pathogens appear to contribute significantly to the intensity of trachoma and to the lesions that impair vision.

Methods of intervention

Chemotherapy

In communities with severe blinding trachoma, the objectives of chemotherapy are:

— to reduce the inflammation in active trachoma in order to reduce the incidence of blinding complications;
— to decrease the transmission of infection.

Sulfonamides, tetracyclines, erythromycin and its derivatives and rifampicin are known to be effective in the treatment of trachoma. Topical

---

[1] Dawson CR, Jones BR, Tarizzo ML. *Guide to trachoma control in programmes for the prevention of blindness.* Geneva, World Health Organization, 1981.

tetracyclines (eye ointments or suspensions) are currently recommended for large-scale treatment, but the development of long-acting oral antibiotics may lead to a significant improvement in community-based treatment.

Trachoma control programmes are based on antibiotic treatment of the whole community, particularly of all children. This "mass therapy" lowers the prevalence of infection and reduces the risk of reinfection. Individual treatment of active cases, even with highly effective antibiotics, is often relatively ineffective because of rapid reinfection. Initial intensive large-scale treatment lowers the prevalence of active trachoma and reduces the ocular reservoir of *Chlamydia* in the population. It should be followed by intermittent, family-based topical treatment to control further eye-to-eye transmission. Such family-based treatment with topically applied antibiotics depends on the local availability of economical and effective drug preparations and on vigorous health education to promote the cleanliness of young children and environmental hygiene, e.g. latrines.

At present, chemotherapy with oral antibiotics is recommended only on a selective basis for severe cases in communities with a high incidence of trachoma (see Table 2).

Treatment with antibiotic ointment, however, involves several problems: eye ointments may be difficult for untrained people to apply; ointments cause blurring of vision; twice-daily dosage is needed for prolonged periods and, even when well monitored, ointment treatment is only partially effective. Moreover, mass treatment with ointment has often been carried out in school populations, which does not affect the reservoir of infection in children aged 1–5 years.

Table 2 summarizes existing strategies for the treatment and control of trachoma.

Treatment with oral antibiotics has been highly effective against trachoma. Oral sulfonamides were once used extensively but had too many unwanted side-effects; oral tetracyclines, particularly long-acting ones, have been effective for mass treatment of older children but cannot be used in children under 7 years of age, the group with the highest rates of active disease; erythromycin is also effective orally but must be given twice daily; rifampicin is reserved primarily for the treatment of tuberculosis and must also be used twice daily.

Oral forms of new erythromycin derivatives have a prolonged period of effectiveness and are now used for the treatment of genital chlamydial infections. These and other new antibiotics may offer a substantial improvement in the treatment of trachoma, but their use will be subject to availability, cost and the experience achieved during full-scale clinical trials.

Table 2. Treatment and control of trachoma

Percentage of children, 1–10 years old, with trachoma	Basic treatment	Additional treatment	Eye health promotion
TF[a]: 20% or more **or** TI[b]: 5% or more	Mass topical antibiotic treatment	Selective systemic antibiotic treatment of severe cases	Improvements in personal hygiene and community sanitation, including: fly control; improvement of community water supplies and waste disposal; distribution of antibiotic ointment during annual outbreaks of purulent conjunctivitis
TF: 5% to 20%	Mass or individual/family topical antibiotic treatment	As above	As above
TF: Less than 5%	Individual topical antibiotic treatment	Not indicated	Case-finding among family members and close contacts

[a] TF = trachomatous inflammation, follicular (see p. 42).
[b] TI = trachomatous inflammation, intense (see p. 42).

Surgical correction of trichiasis and entropion

The correction of lid deformities and inturned eyelashes has an immediate impact in preventing blindness. A simple procedure that can be carried out in affected communities has been described (Reacher, Foster & Huber, 1993). Surgical programmes may still be required where active trachoma is no longer a problem but where trachomatous scarring continues to evolve and to cause lid deformities and visual loss.

Action at various levels

Primary level

The application of antibiotics to the eye can often be carried out, after simple training, by local health workers with few, if any, formal qualifications. In the long run, most topical antibiotic treatment must be carried out by the affected people themselves. Treatment programmes should also be accompanied by active programmes of health education that emphasize the daily washing of young children and the use of latrines. Other sanitary measures include the provision of clean water, reduction of household crowding and elimination of the breeding sites of eye-seeking flies.

Secondary level

Eyelid surgery that is provided in the community itself is essential to block the route to blindness from chronic trachoma. This surgery can be provided by either health centres or mobile teams. Experience has shown that selected and appropriately trained medical auxiliaries can provide most of the lid surgery needed.

Once the backlog of trichiasis and entropion has been treated, there will be a continuing need for surgery on a lesser scale because cases of potentially blinding lid distortion will continue to arise long after the infective stages of trachoma have been controlled. In severely affected communities, periodic surveillance and the provision of lid surgery will be required for many years.

Organizational aspects

Planning and integration

The primary objective of public health programmes for the control of trachoma is the prevention of blindness. Such programmes should be designed and implemented as an integral part of activities aimed at controlling blindness from other major causes. Once control of blinding trachoma has been achieved, surveillance should be maintained to detect the occurrence of potentially blinding trachoma.

Control programmes should be focused on communities with a substantial prevalence of blinding trachoma, as indicated by the presence of:

— corneal blindness;
— potentially blinding trachomatous trichiasis and entropion;
— moderate and severe trachomatous inflammation.

Preliminary prevalence surveys can identify communities with blinding trachoma, i.e. the presence of people with severe visual loss due to corneal opacity and a high prevalence of follicular or intense trachoma and trichiasis or entropion. Surveys should also assess blindness rates as well as other potential causes of blindness in the community.

Training

Effective control of blinding trachoma can be achieved by the introduction of relatively simple measures which can be implemented by appropri-

46

ately trained health personnel, including auxiliary health workers. Training of personnel is therefore an essential part of trachoma control. The development of simplified procedures for the assessment of trachoma and its complications and for the provision of surgery for trichiasis and entropion has allowed for greater reliance on auxiliary personnel for the prevention and control of trachoma (see, e.g., *Primary health care level management of trachoma*; *Achieving community support for trachoma control*).

Evaluation

The selection of target populations is a critical first step in trachoma control. Follow-up assessments are then necessary to evaluate the effectiveness of the intervention. The needs of each community change continuously and must be reviewed at regular intervals. Antibiotic treatment and economic development may substantially and rapidly reduce the prevalence of disease. On the other hand, in communities with a substantial amount of potentially disabling scarring, new cases of trichiasis and entropion will continue to appear and continuing surveillance will be necessary for many years after active inflammatory trachoma has been controlled.

Recommendations for community-based trachoma control

Community-oriented treatment of trachoma should aim at decreasing the intensity of the disease and reducing the reservoir of infection, particularly in children. The identification and correction of deformed eyelids are also essential components in the prevention of blindness due to trachoma.

Community and social development

The provision of clean water for domestic use, reduction of household crowding, the elimination of the breeding sites of eye-seeking flies and improved personal hygiene all help to reduce the intensity of inflammation due to trachoma. Health education is an essential tool in achieving these changes.

Antimicrobial therapy

The mass application of a topical antibiotic (usually a tetracycline) may be supplemented by oral antibiotics (see Table 2).

Lid surgery

Surgical intervention for deformed eyelids and inturned eyelashes has an immediate effect in preventing blindness and includes the following components:

- *Case-finding*
  - identification of affected people in the community by local health workers or others;
  - screening of the population by specially trained personnel.
- *Provision of corrective surgery*
  - referral to the nearest district hospital or secondary centre where lid surgery is available;
  - use of mobile teams for case-finding and surgery every 6–12 months.

Temporary measures that can be used if surgery is not immediately available include the periodic removal of lashes that are irritating or damaging the cornea and the application of tetracycline or other antibiotic ointment twice daily.

Blinding malnutrition

Present state of knowledge

Blinding malnutrition (xerophthalmia, keratomalacia) is the result of a prolonged lack of vitamin A, often combined with general malnutrition and deprivation. Before this blinding stage (obvious from the presence of eye signs) is reached, subclinical vitamin A deficiency contributes to an increased severity of certain infections and an increased risk of dying from them.

Vitamin A is essential for many bodily functions, including vision, cellular integrity, immune competence and growth. Vitamin A deficiency, therefore, is a systemic disease that affects cells and tissues throughout the body. The most specific and recognized effects of severe vitamin A deficiency involve the eye.

Vitamin A is necessary for synthesis of the photosensitive pigments of retinal cells and for normal differentiation of mucus-secreting epithelial structures. Severe deficiency results in night blindness, xerosis and keratinization of the conjunctiva and cornea, and ultimately corneal ulceration and liquefactive necrosis.

Multiple factors affect an individual's vitamin A status. One of the most important is adequate intake of vitamin A and provitamin A (retinol and carotenoids with vitamin A activity, respectively). The recommended intake is at least 180–450 µg of retinol or retinol equivalents (RE) per day, depending on age, sex and physiological status.[1] Populations at risk of blinding malnutrition generally receive most of their vitamin A from carotenoid-containing yellow and green fruits and vegetables. Such foods are often available only seasonally; thus, the dietary intake must be several times the daily requirement to ensure the build-up of adequate body stores of vitamin A to carry through periods when the availability and consumption of vitamin A and provitamin A are low.

---

[1] Sommer A. *Vitamin A deficiency and its consequences: a field guide to detection and control*, 3rd ed. Geneva, World Health Organization, 1995.

Diarrhoea, worm infestations and other intestinal disorders impair vitamin A absorption, while measles, respiratory tract infections and other febrile illnesses increase metabolic demands and often interfere with normal appetite. Protein–energy malnutrition is an added burden that interferes with the absorption, storage and utilization of vitamin A. Where these aggravating factors are common, the dietary requirements for vitamin A are increased. In some instances, corneal destruction due to malnutrition may be exacerbated by secondary bacterial infections that are frequently associated with poor personal hygiene.

Epidemiology

Blindness due to malnutrition can occur at any age. The various contributory factors (e.g. frequent diarrhoea, measles, other febrile illnesses and protein–energy malnutrition) occur most frequently among young children of disadvantaged communities. Such children, therefore, are at the highest risk for xerophthalmia. Severe, blinding corneal destruction (keratomalacia) is a disease largely limited to the first 5 years of life, and is especially prevalent among those aged 6–36 months. The younger the child and the more severe the disease, the higher is the associated mortality. A majority of patients with keratomalacia who do not receive medical attention probably die.

Blinding malnutrition is endemic in much of Africa and South and East Asia with scattered foci in Central and South America, the Eastern Mediterranean and the Western Pacific. Most childhood blindness in Africa, and much of that occurring in other endemic areas, is secondary to infection with measles, which precipitates acute, severe, clinical vitamin A deficiency among children with mildly to moderately poor vitamin A and protein status.

Since the factors responsible for vitamin A deficiency are generally shared by other members of the household and neighbourhood, patients with xerophthalmia have a tendency to be found clustered within discrete areas. The presence of clinically evident vitamin A deficiency therefore identifies an area as one where there is likely to be subclinical vitamin A deficiency in the surrounding population.

Programmes of prophylactic vitamin A administration and efforts to improve socioeconomic conditions in some endemic countries have successfully reduced the prevalence of severe vitamin A deficiency and blinding malnutrition. Subclinical vitamin A deficiency, however, remains an important public health problem contributing to childhood morbidity and mortality. Even now it is likely that, globally, at least one-quarter of a million patients develop keratomalacia annually, more than half of whom probably die. Perhaps 10 times as many children as those with xerophthalmia, who are estimated to number about 14 million, are sub-clinically vitamin A deficient. Their risk of dying is increased by 23–30% when they contract common childhood infections such as diarrhoea and measles.

In 1996, WHO identified 76 countries with a significant public health problem of vitamin A deficiency.[1]

Symptoms and diagnosis

Uncomplicated, gradual vitamin A depletion results in changes of increasing severity in cells and organs throughout the body. The respiratory system, urinary tract, the intestinal epithelium and components of the immune system (i.e. the body's general defences against disease) are all probably affected before the deficiency is clinically observable. Moreover, changes in ocular tissue occur only relatively late in the progression of clinical vitamin A deficiency.

Night blindness is the earliest symptom that is readily detected, i.e. the affected child has difficulty seeing under reduced levels of light. Among populations in which vitamin A deficiency is endemic, a recent history of night blindness in a young child almost invariably indicates vitamin A deficiency. In such populations, specific terms usually exist to describe the condition (e.g. "chicken eyes").

As vitamin A deficiency advances, the conjunctiva becomes affected by a keratinizing metaplasia that is the result of the loss of goblet cells and the formation of a granular layer of unwettable epithelial cells. This is known as conjunctival xerosis, apparent as an oval or triangular patch in the temporal quadrant of the conjunctiva. With a more severe deficiency, the conjunctival involvement is more extensive and may extend to the nasal quadrant.

When desquamated keratin and bacteria accumulate on the dry conjunctival surface, appearing as foamy or cheesy material, the lesion is known as a Bitot's spot. Bitot's spots in preschool-aged children usually indicate vitamin A deficiency and respond to treatment with vitamin A. In children of school age, these spots are often the inactive sequelae of earlier disease and may be less responsive to vitamin A treatment. In older individuals, Bitot's spots may be due to causes other than vitamin A deficiency and a careful history is needed to reveal their etiology.

Corneal changes begin early in clinical vitamin A deficiency, about the time that night blindness is noted but before conjunctival xerosis is

---

[1] *Indicators for assessing vitamin A deficiency and their application in monitoring and evaluating intervention programmes.* Geneva, World Health Organization, 1996 (unpublished document WHO/NUT/96.10; available on request from Division of Food and Nutrition, World Health Organization, 1211 Geneva 27, Switzerland).

evident. These early changes cannot be seen by the unaided eye. They consist of superficial punctate lesions of the lower nasal quadrant of the cornea that can be detected only by a slit-lamp and that spread upward with increasingly severe disease.

Corneal xerosis begins as a hazy, dry, non-wettable area in the inferior part of the cornea. With more severe deficiency the changes become more striking and cover a larger part of the corneal surface. Plaques of keratinized cells resembling Bitot's spots occasionally form on the corneal surface.

The foregoing abnormalities are reversible by treatment with vitamin A for 2–5 days, and the cornea regains a normal appearance in 1–2 weeks. Once loss of corneal stroma occurs, however, the result is permanent structural damage and scarring. The mildest form of stromal loss is one or more small, circular or oval, sharply demarcated corneal ulcers of varying depth. Perforating ulcers are usually plugged with iris (adherent leukoma), which preserves the basic integrity of the eye. Prompt treatment of mild stromal loss results in a small peripheral scar but retention of good vision.

Focal areas of corneal necrosis (keratomalacia) begin as opaque, bulging masses of the corneal surface that rapidly progress in size. These lesions heal as dense, white, adherent leukomas. When less than one-third of the corneal surface is involved, useful vision is preserved. More extensive corneal involvement may result in generalized liquefactive necrosis, extrusion of intraocular contents and loss of the globe. Prompt therapy may preserve the other eye.

Xerophthalmia does not always occur in the sequence outlined above. Acute decompensation of borderline vitamin A deficiency, which sometimes occurs in patients with febrile conditions, especially measles, may result in rapid and extensive corneal destruction in eyes that had previously appeared normal. A similar response may result from feeding a diet lacking vitamin A but rich in energy and protein to severely malnourished children who may be subclinically vitamin A deficient. Accelerated growth resulting from an improved protein status can rapidly exhaust meagre vitamin A reserves. Even with gradual vitamin A depletion, parents may be unaware of the onset of the night blindness and inflammation that commonly accompany corneal ulceration and necrosis and that may mask conjunctival xerosis.

Methods of intervention

Treatment

Prompt treatment of children with xerophthalmia, or any corneal ulceration due to vitamin A deficiency, with high doses of vitamin A is essential. The preferred route of administration is oral because it is safe and effective in most cases. The age-specific treatment schedule is given in Table 3.

The uncommon instances when an intramuscular route of administration may be necessary include treatment of children who are unable to swallow because of severe stomatitis or persistent vomiting as well as those with severe malabsorption syndromes. In these instances, intramuscular injections of 55 mg (100 000 IU) of water-miscible retinyl palmitate should be substituted for the first oral dose for children over 1 year of age. For children 6–12 months of age the dose should be reduced by half, and for those under 6 months by three-quarters. In no circumstance should oil-based injections be used to treat xerophthalmia: these preparations are ineffective in saving sight and life.

Because of the demonstrated association between the onset of xerophthalmia and frequent and persistent diarrhoea, protein–energy malnutrition, measles and other febrile infections, including pneumonia, children residing in areas of endemic vitamin A deficiency should receive vitamin A supplements as part of disease-specific case management. Case-management schedules are presented in Table 4.

Prevention

Before instituting a prophylaxis programme, it is necessary to determine whether, where and among whom endemic vitamin A deficiency and blinding malnutrition are important public health problems. Knowledge of breast-feeding, and of dietary and disease patterns that might contribute to vitamin A deficiency should be obtained. The availability and consumption of food sources of vitamin A and provitamin A by vulnerable groups should be assessed. This information, combined with knowledge of other demographic and ecological risk factors as well as culturally specific eating habits, is useful to define populations at risk where definitive biochemical and clinical surveys can be conducted. Biochemical and clinical data can be compared with reference criteria established by WHO[1] to determine whether vitamin A deficiency poses a problem of public health importance.

Prevention of blinding malnutrition takes two forms: increasing vitamin A intake and reducing the prevalence and severity of factors that contribute to its occurrence, such as measles, frequent diarrhoea, respiratory infections and protein–energy malnutrition. Of these, measles is likely to be the most readily preventable. An effective measles immunization programme

---

[1] Sommer A. *Vitamin A deficiency and its consequences: a field guide to detection and control,* 3rd ed. Geneva, World Health Organization, 1995:34.

Table 3. Treatment schedule for xerophthalmia

Timing	Dosage by mouth[a]
Immediately on diagnosis (by age):	
<6 months	27.5 mg retinyl palmitate (50 000 IU)
6–12 months	55 mg retinyl palmitate (100 000 IU)
>12 months	110 mg retinyl palmitate (200 000 IU)
Next day	Same age-specific dosage
If clinical deterioration occurs or, when possible, 1–4 weeks later	Same age-specific dosage

[a] Intramuscular injection of water-miscible retinyl palmitate at half these dosages can be substituted in rare instances when swallowing is severely impaired, vomiting is persistent or severe malabsorption prevents an adequate response.

Table 4. Case-management schedules for areas with endemic vitamin A deficiency

Disease	Dosage by mouth	Timing
Measles (by 'age):		
<12 months	55 mg retinyl palmitate (100 000 IU)	On diagnosis and a second dose the next day
≥12 months	110 mg retinyl palmitate (200 000 IU)	Same schedule
Severe protein–energy malnutrition	Same age-specific dosage	Once with close supervision. If condition worsens give second dose
Persistent diarrhoea	Same age-specific dosage	Once per episode with at least a 1-month interval between doses
Other prolonged febrile illnesses/ conditions	Same age-specific dosage	Once per episode with at least a 1-month interval between doses

in an area of vitamin A deficiency is likely to prevent most related blindness and death. Adequate attention should be given to contributory environmental and dietary factors in order to achieve a sustainable solution to vitamin A deficiency.

The most direct, effective and sustainable solution is ensuring that children consume food with adequate quantities of vitamin A and other essential micronutrients, as well as protein and calories. Mothers should be encouraged to breast-feed exclusively (without giving additional water) until babies reach 4–6 months of age, since breast milk generally is adequate for this period and is safe and protective. By 6 months of age, provitamin A-rich foods, such as mashed cooked carrot or yellow sweet potato, mango and papaya in small amounts (2–3 spoonsful daily) should begin to complement breast-feeding. Dark-green leafy vegetables (3–4 spoonsful) should be added to the diet at least three times weekly, along with adequate calories and protein from staple foods, by 1 year of age, while continuing breast-feeding. Few families of high-risk communities can afford foods rich in the more easily absorbed preformed vitamin, such as eggs, fish and animal liver, and whole-milk dairy products. Breast milk contains sufficient fat to facilitate the absorption of vitamin A, but adding a small amount of fat or oil to lipid-poor, post-weaning diets will improve absorption. Cooking and shredding or mashing vitamin A-containing vegetables promotes absorption, but prolonged overcooking is destructive of the vitamin.

Where foods rich in vitamin A and provitamin A are inexpensive and already available, nutritional education programmes are needed to create an awareness of their value, stimulate demand for them and encourage consumption. Where such foods are expensive or unavailable, the introduction or stimulation of their home-provisioning through gardening may prove feasible; between a quarter and a half a mango or papaya, or half a cup of dark-green leafy vegetable, will supply the daily vitamin A requirement of most young children. Where products in the garden are highly seasonal (e.g. mangoes and some green leaves) ways of preserving them across seasons, such as solar drying, should be sought.

Green leafy vegetables prepared for young children should be lightly boiled and drained; the excess water should be discarded, as it may contain unwanted soluble substances such as oxalates, cyanates and poly-phenols that interfere with the absorption of iron and other micro-nutrients that frequently are also in short supply. Green leafy vegetables are more likely to be acceptable to children if they are first strained to remove excess fibre or cut into small pieces and thoroughly mixed into the staple food (e.g. rice, maize gruel).

Where high-risk groups consume little fat or oils, a small amount should be mixed into the diet to enhance vitamin A absorption.

Vitamin A fortification of foodstuffs—including cereals, fats and oils, and condiments—that are commonly consumed has also been a successful strategy to increase vitamin A intake in some situations.

Periodic oral administration of large doses of vitamin A is a direct short-term method of preventing vitamin A deficiency in high-risk populations. Supplements should be given to malnourished mothers in endemically deficient areas within 1 month of delivery (a single dose of 200 000 IU retinyl palmitate) and to infants and children as indicated in Table 5. Giving vitamin A supplements directly to mothers will improve their vitamin A status, that of their breast milk and that of their nursing infant.

Women of childbearing age, however, should not be given large doses of supplemental vitamin A because these can be teratogenic if taken during the early part of pregnancy. Preferably, fertile women should obtain their vitamin A requirements through food. Where this cannot be accomplished, controlled administration of doses not exceeding 10 000 IU daily is safe.

Action at various levels

Primary level

Where xerophthalmia is known to be a major public health problem, consideration should be given to instituting immediate, controlled, generalized prophylaxis by periodically administering large doses of vitamin A to the population at risk (see Table 5). However, the programme should include a definite plan to replace supplementation within a specified time period by a more sustainable solution. The vitamin supplements should be administered by village or urban primary health care workers utilizing existing infrastructures such as clinics or community weighing

Table 5. Vitamin A prophylaxis schedule for areas of endemic vitamin A deficiency

Group	Dosage by mouth	Timing
Infants:		
<6 months	27.5 mg retinyl palmitate (50 000 IU)	Once to those not being breast-fed
6–12 months	55 mg retinyl palmitate (100 000 IU)	Once
Children > 12 months	110 mg retinyl palmitate (200 000 IU)	Every 4–6 months until they are receiving adequate dietary sources
Lactating women within 4 weeks of delivery	110 mg retinyl palmitate (200 000 IU)	Once within 1 month (or 2 months at most) of giving birth
Fertile women at other times, including pregnancy and lactation	Not to exceed 5.5 mg retinyl palmitate (10 000 IU)	Daily, at most

stations in which there is periodic and routine contact with preschool-aged children and their mothers.

In addition to routine distribution of vitamin A supplements, the primary health care worker should know how to recognize xerophthalmia and should examine all children, particularly those who are malnourished or sick, for this condition (i.e. enquiring about the presence of night blindness and looking for evidence of Bitot's spots and corneal xerosis and ulceration).

Children with xerophthalmia or any of the major contributory conditions (e.g. diarrhoea, respiratory tract infection, measles, protein–energy malnutrition) should receive oral vitamin A as shown in Tables 3 and 4, in addition to therapy for the primary illness. Children who fail to respond to therapy should be referred to a secondary facility, as should any children with corneal ulceration or necrosis.

To facilitate the process leading to sustainable elimination of vitamin A deficiency, primary health care workers should be familiar with locally available low-cost sources of vitamin A that are acceptable for feeding young children. Mothers should be encouraged to feed children these foods frequently, especially children who are recovering from illness. Local community organizations such as schoolteachers and women's groups can expand the outreach of the primary health care worker in this regard.

Because vitamin A deficiency clusters in families and neighbourhoods, families of affected children and their neighbours—and, if at all possible, the rest of the village—should be made aware of the potential seriousness of the problem and the ease with which it can be prevented. They should be provided with specific instructions about which locally available foods to feed their children and how best to prepare them. The awareness and support of local political and community leaders can enhance such efforts. To extend the impact of local efforts, use can be made of the communications media.

Secondary level

Where village-level workers are not available, primary xerophthalmia control is provided by static centres (health posts, clinics, hospitals, etc.). For the most part, these reach only children presenting themselves at the facility. Since vitamin A deficiency clusters in communities, a modest outreach programme to affected communities can be a cost-effective means of dealing with the problem. Staff of static centres can visit the neighbourhoods from which the xerophthalmia cases arise, administer vitamin A to all preschool-aged children (see Table 5), and provide nutritional education to their families. Among cultures that readily recognize night blindness, teachers can instruct schoolchildren to report the condition when present among younger siblings. Staff of district or sub-district centres should respond to a positive report from localities in exactly the same way as to a self-referred patient.

Static centres often have better trained staff, more plentiful medical supplies and inpatient facilities. They are therefore better able to handle cases of corneal ulceration and necrosis (and the severe illnesses commonly accompanying them) than are village-level workers. Their personnel may also be able to supervise primary health care workers and provide them with refresher courses, feedback and encouragement.

Primary- and secondary-level facilities should ensure the ready availability of a high-potency vitamin A preparation at all centres.

Tertiary level

There is little need for sophisticated, tertiary-level care in the treatment of blinding malnutrition. Prompt vitamin A therapy will usually preserve useful vision whenever that is still possible. Those blinded by xerophthalmia rarely benefit from corneal transplantation. In a few cases an optical iridectomy may restore some vision.

Organizational aspects

Planning and integration

Central staff must first determine, through a systematic assessment, whether vitamin A deficiency, including blinding malnutrition, is an important problem, in which areas it is most severe and the reasons for its presence. An appropriate intervention strategy will reflect this information, the available resources and the existing community health care delivery systems that may be useful.

Some strategies, like the provision of a fortified diet, are necessarily centralized and often national in character. Implementation requires decisions concerning the appropriate foodstuffs or seasonings and the level of fortification, the passage of relevant legislation or regulations and the maintenance of strict quality monitoring of the final product, both as it leaves the factory and at the periphery since transport and storage may affect the stability of its ingredients. Community awareness of the need to consume fortified products should be created, particularly where a choice exists for a similar but unfortified product at a slightly lower price.

The central level is often responsible for the preparation of nutritional education campaigns (as well as the messages or "spots" for use by radio, television and cinemas and the posters, flip-charts and other visual aids required by workers at the peripheral level). It is important for the nutritional information that is distributed to be flexible, so that local variation in available vitamin A-rich food sources and their preparation, use and preservation can be accommodated.

Training

All levels of health personnel should be properly informed about blinding malnutrition and its prevention. The specific content of training will depend, of course, on the nature of the individual's involvement with the disease. Physicians, medical officers and graduate nurses often represent the principal source of information, supervision and motivation at the secondary and tertiary levels. Therefore, they need to be familiar with all aspects of the problem. For example, ophthalmologists need to appreciate the importance to child health and survival of correcting even subclinical vitamin A deficiency. Brief, periodic refresher courses will stimulate their interest and maintain their competence.

A more simplified, practical curriculum is appropriate for the training of primary health care workers. Emphasis should be placed on the seriousness of the problem, particularly the fact that it arises from faulty dietary practices (e.g. lack of breast-feeding) and that children with protein–energy malnutrition, diarrhoea, respiratory tract infections, measles or any severe illness are at a high risk of nutritionally engendered blindness, as are apparently healthy children living in the immediate vicinity of a patient with active xerophthalmia. Workers should be able to recognize, though not necessarily classify, night blindness, Bitot's spots, corneal ulcers and necrosis, understand the need for prompt, therapeutic doses of vitamin A and correction of the underlying systemic diseases, and know how to refer children with severe disease (inflamed, ulcerated eyes) to secondary facilities after initiating emergency large-dose therapy. Supervision, feedback and periodic retraining by higher-level medical personnel or specialized primary eye care workers are essential for maintaining motivation and competence.

Primary health care workers should be capable of providing nutritional education in villages by counselling the families and neighbours of affected children. Regular village nutritional education campaigns, however, are often delegated to specialized nutrition or general health education personnel. In either instance, methods for increasing vitamin A intake should be provided in the context of general dietary improvement and the prevention of malnutrition and infectious diseases.

Often, local traditional midwives can be effectively incorporated into the system by training them to carry out specific supportive tasks under the control of the primary health care worker. For example, they could supply to malnourished mothers, at the time of childbirth, a high-dose vitamin A supplement provided by the health worker.

Training aids and clinical recognition cards,[1] already available through WHO and other agencies, may prove useful, but should be tailored to local needs.

Evaluation

Evaluation should be an integral part of any programme. Some methods are extremely simple, such as monitoring the number of vitamin A capsules or measles vaccine doses distributed, but these do not reveal whether vitamin A-deficient mothers or children in fact received them. For more definitive assessment, special recording procedures should be established at the household or family level. Spot checks of family health cards retained in households can then establish the proportion of target mothers and children who actually received the agent. Both of these methods assess the *process*. To assess *outcome*, i.e. whether the programme reduces the number of children with xerophthalmia or who become blind, clinical information must be collected. One simple method is to establish and periodically review a standardized recording system for xerophthalmia cases encountered by selected village health workers, and in sentinel clinics and hospitals operating in high-risk areas. More definitive assessment requires periodic examination of a random sample of all preschool-aged children residing in such areas. WHO has developed survey forms for this purpose.[1] As a general rule, individuals directly responsible for implementing a programme should not be the same as those evaluating it, but close coordination between the two is essential, because evaluation should also indicate methods by which the programme can be improved.

---

[1] Available on request from Division of Food and Nutrition, World Health Organization, 1211 Geneva 27, Switzerland.

Onchocerciasis

Present state of knowledge

General aspects and epidemiology

Onchocerciasis is a blinding parasitic disease caused by a filarial worm, *Onchocerca volvulus*, which is transmitted from person to person by the bite of blackflies of the genus *Simulium*. Nearly 18 million people are affected by the disease, and it is estimated that approximately half a million are severely visually impaired, with an additional 270 000 rendered blind.

Onchocerciasis occurs in 27 countries in tropical Africa, all lying between latitudes 12°N and 15°S. It is also found in isolated foci in six countries in Central and South America and affects a limited number of people in the Republic of Yemen.

The final host is human beings, in whom the adult forms of the parasite live in either an encapsulated or a free state. The female worm releases embryos, or microfilariae, which invade the tissues and involve not only the skin and eye, where their presence is very easy to demonstrate, but also the internal organs.

Microfilariae are ingested by female blackflies when they bite and take their blood meal from an infected person. The microfilariae develop in the fly for an average of 7 days until they attain the infective form which reenters a human host when the fly feeds again. These infective larvae eventually develop into adult male and female worms, which in some cases form easily recognized nodules under the skin. The adult female is capable, after fertilization, of releasing myriads of microfilarial embryos which can initiate a new cycle of infection. The average life-span of the adult parasite is about 10 years, with a maximum of 15 years.

The blackfly vector lives near rivers, where it lays its eggs in fast-running water. In West Africa, it is known to fly more than 500 kilometres, assisted by monsoon winds, and to colonize far-off rivers. The blackfly feeds during the daytime. Its bites are a source of substantial discomfort, as the number of bites per person per day may reach several thousand.

The pattern and severity of the disease vary from one geographical area to another, depending on the intensity of transmission and differences in the parasite and its vector.

Many African villages close to large breeding sites of *Simulium damnosum* carry the social burden of a large blind population. Under these conditions, adolescents and young adults in the village tend to migrate to seek work elsewhere, and the entire community may disintegrate, with abandonment of the village.

In many onchocerciasis-endemic areas of West Africa, vast areas of cultivable land alongside rivers are uninhabited. In areas with high rates of microfilarial transmission, and hence a large proportion of disabled persons, a population density of less than 50 persons per square kilometre constitutes a critical threshold for total desertion of the land.

The manifestations of onchocerciasis

Onchocerciasis is a cumulative parasitosis. In general, cutaneous and ocular manifestations in a given individual increase with the number of bites and with the number of parasites in the skin. In hyperendemic areas, the disease usually becomes clinically apparent in young adults. The main signs are the presence of palpable subcutaneous nodules, itching and a fine papular rash, which is easily overlooked. In later stages there is usually atrophy of the skin and there are also changes in pigmentation.

Onchocercal involvement of the eye causes lacrimation, photophobia and itching. Pain may result from iritis and glaucoma. Usually, however, the disease progresses insidiously over several decades. Night blindness and narrowing of the visual field commonly occur at an early stage of the disease. Serious impairment of vision often develops more rapidly in the late and irreversible stages of the disease.

The early onchocercal corneal manifestation, punctate keratitis, is reversible. However, the more severe chronic sclerosing keratitis, which is painless, constitutes an important cause of permanent visual loss, as do lesions in the retina and optic nerve.

Ocular lesions are the most disabling manifestation of the disease. In some African savannah villages the prevalence of onchocercal blindness may be as high as 10% of the total population, and severe eye complications may be present in more than 50% of the adults.

Diagnosis

Onchocerciasis is most easily diagnosed by the skin snip technique, which is an easy and safe test that can be performed by a laboratory auxiliary worker. The test provides evidence of the parasite in the skin, and counting the parasites gives a quantitative evaluation of the cutaneous parasite density. An immunodiagnostic test is in the developmental stage and is expected to complement the skin snip test in due course.

Methods of intervention

The goal of onchocerciasis treatment is elimination of the microfilariae and adult worms of *Onchocerca volvulus* from patients. Two methods of intervention can be employed. The first is directed against the vector—the blackfly—with larvicide, and the second is directed against the parasite in humans by chemotherapy.

Larvicide can be particularly effective against the vector when applied over a large enough area in fast-flowing rivers where breeding sites are located. This approach has been applied successfully in the Onchocerciasis Control Programme area in West Africa, which covers 650 000 square kilometres in the seven original countries of the programme. In this area, the breeding sites of the vector have been sprayed regularly for a period of 14 to 15 years with fixed-wing aircraft and helicopters in order to interrupt the transmission of infection. Such an approach entails sophisticated logistics and organization, is expensive and cannot be applied in all endemic countries.

The use of chemotherapy to treat onchocerciasis in the past was unpopular because the existing drugs, diethylcarbamazine and suramin, caused severe and unacceptable side-effects. Another drug (ivermectin) has been developed which is an effective long-acting microfilaricide suitable for large-scale treatment in endemic countries. Ivermectin is provided free of charge under the trade name Mectizan by the pharmaceutical firm Merck & Co. to all endemic countries that have set up onchocerciasis control programmes.

At present, ivermectin distribution to control onchocerciasis is the method of intervention being applied in all endemic countries outside the area of the Onchocerciasis Control Programme in West Africa. Ivermectin is given once a year to all those who are eligible to take it. As onchocerciasis occurs mainly in rural areas, which often have poorly accessible roads and lack medical facilities, ivermectin distribution to the needy entails much planning and organization and is associated with some inevitable costs. Typical dosages for ivermectin are given in Table 6.

The following groups are excluded from treatment:

— children less than 5 years old, or less than 15 kg in weight or 95 cm in height;
— pregnant women;

Table 6. Treatment of onchocerciasis with ivermectin

Weight in kg	Height in cm	Dosage (6-mg tablets)
15–24	90–119	1/2
25–44	120–140	1
45–64	141–158	1–1/2
65–85	>158	2

— mothers who are breast-feeding babies less than 1 week old;
— people with disease of the central nervous system;
— severely ill people.

Action at various levels

Primary level

Where onchocerciasis is hyperendemic, the aim of intervention is to distribute ivermectin to the entire eligible population in the community. To administer treatment cost-effectively, village health workers are used to establish a register of the people in a target village and to administer the requisite quantity of the drug to individuals according to weight or height. These health workers keep a tally of the number of tablets they use in treating the community. In addition, they can treat any mild adverse reactions and refer severe reactions to the nearest health centre for management.

In areas where onchocerciasis is only hypoendemic, ivermectin can be made available in health centres and people made aware of its availability and encouraged to attend health centres for treatment.

Secondary level

Ivermectin tablets can be made available in fixed health institutions where patients presenting with signs and symptoms of onchocerciasis are treated.

Personnel at district hospitals also usually supervise the activities of staff at the primary level and give managerial and organizational support. They can conduct periodic training of health staff and village health workers who are distributing ivermectin in selected communities.

Tertiary level

Ivermectin tablets can be made available at tertiary centres so that patients presenting with signs and symptoms of onchocerciasis can be treated.

As at the secondary level, personnel at the tertiary level will be expected to give managerial and organizational support, in this case to both secondary and primary levels. Ordering ivermectin tablets and distributing them to the districts—and eventually to the periphery—is the responsibility of tertiary-level management. Evaluation of ivermectin distribution is also initiated at the tertiary level.

Organizational aspects

Planning and integration

The control of onchocerciasis by ivermectin distribution requires good planning and organization. A national coordinator should be appointed, who would be responsible for the initial central planning and organization. However, it is essential to involve the primary health care system and foster community participation right from the beginning, to ensure the sustainability of ivermectin distribution and to avoid the creation of a vertical programme.

The objective of onchocerciasis control by ivermectin distribution is to eliminate onchocerciasis as a public health problem. The strategies involved are therefore aimed primarily at the community and not at the individual patient. The aim should be to distribute ivermectin to all who are eligible to take it; if it is to be sustainable, the method employed should be cost-effective as well as affordable.

Programmes to control onchocerciasis by ivermectin distribution should include the following elements:

— rapid epidemiological mapping to determine the distribution and severity of onchocerciasis in the country;
— selection of communities that need to be treated through rapid epidemiological assessment surveys;
— training of health personnel and primary health care workers;
— development of health education materials and execution of health education and public awareness campaigns with emphasis on community participation;
— choice and planning of methods of distribution;
— execution of distribution activities;
— monitoring and evaluation of the intervention.

Training

Training should be undertaken at all levels. At the tertiary and secondary levels, it should cover the epidemiology, manifestations and diagnosis of onchocerciasis (including rapid epidemiological assessment surveys, i.e. nodule palpation of adult males aged at least 20 years—a sample size of 50 in a community of 300 or more people is sufficient), and treatment strategies, including record-keeping. The aim should be to create managers and trainers.

At the district level, primary health care staff should receive similar training adapted to their level of expertise. Primary health care staff should be trained and employed to carry out ivermectin distribution. There should be emphasis on census-taking, nodule palpation, modalities of treatment, treatment dosage, exclusion criteria, record-keeping of treatment and tablets, and management of adverse reactions.

At the village level, the community should identify a village health worker who will be trained to open a village register, administer the correct dosage of ivermectin to all eligible individuals, keep a record of the tablets used, treat mild adverse reactions and recognize serious reactions for referral to the nearest health centre.

Monitoring

Monitoring at all levels is an essential part of ivermectin distribution to control onchocerciasis. Primary health care personnel will monitor the activities of village health workers, and secondary- and possibly also tertiary-level personnel will monitor the work of primary health care personnel, as well as carry out random checking of village health workers.

Evaluation

Indicator communities should be selected to undergo skin-snip testing before the first treatment and at intervals thereafter to enable the impact of the intervention to be assessed.

Sustainability

The success of the control of onchocerciasis will depend on the cost-effectiveness of the ivermectin distribution and on full integration of the distribution into the primary health care system. The ultimate goal of the distribution should be treatment of communities by village health workers, with secondary-level health care staff monitoring and evaluating the distribution as an additional activity carried out in the course of their passage through the village.

Cataract[1]

Present state of knowledge

Description

The loss of vision from cataract is a major cause of blindness in developing countries that can be treated successfully with existing technology. Since the prevalence of cataract rises markedly with age, blindness from cataract in developing countries will increase very rapidly as a result of the expected increase in the number of old people over the next 50 years. Even in areas with blinding diseases such as trachoma and onchocerciasis, cataract is a major cause of blindness.

Cataract is generally defined as an opacity of the crystalline lens of the eye. Minor opacities are extremely common and rarely interfere substantially with vision. More extensive opacities interfere with light passing through the crystalline lens and cause distortion of, or considerable reduction in, the light rays falling on the retina.

About 85% of cataracts are classified as senile, the causes of which are unknown. There are many known causes of cataract, but these account for a relatively small percentage (i.e. about 15%) of the total number of cases. The present understanding of the biochemical and structural events leading to the formation of senile cataract is quite incomplete.

Although not a major cause of vision loss in absolute terms, congenital cataract is of particular importance because it affects infants and young children and therefore, if left untreated, causes lifelong blindness. At the present time these patients are usually treated surgically at tertiary eye care centres, because general anaesthesia is required and the surgical procedures are much more technically demanding than routine surgery for senile cataract. To ensure a good visual outcome, surgery and optical correction should be done as early as possible, preferably before 6 months of age.

---

[1] For a fuller discussion, see *Management of cataract in primary health care services*, 2nd ed. Geneva, World Health Organization, 1996.

In countries where cataract is a major blinding condition and where most of the ophthalmologists' efforts are devoted to cataract surgery, it is essential that the accumulation (backlog) of patients with unoperated cataracts be eliminated as soon as possible. Once an extra effort has been made to eliminate the patient backlog, it is possible to cope with the annual incidence of new cataract cases routinely. The number of people with unoperated cataracts should be estimated, and a time limit—not more than 5–10 years—should be set for elimination of the backlog. Governments and nongovernmental agencies should adopt policies that would encourage and facilitate cataract surgery in rural areas to assist in this effort. If insufficient numbers of ophthalmologists or surgical technicians are nationally available, appropriate personnel should be trained and, in the meantime, other solutions should be explored, such as short-term assistance from international volunteer organizations.

Epidemiology

Magnitude of the problem

Although the biochemistry of cataract formation has been studied extensively, there has been relatively little research on the distribution and probable causes of cataract in human populations. There are three major ways to study the magnitude of the cataract problem: prevalence surveys, blindness registries and model reporting areas, and the number of operations performed.

Prevalence surveys from developing countries indicate that cataract is the greatest cause of severe visual impairment. It accounts for about 50% of blindness, with overall blindness rates due to cataract between 1% and nearly 4% of the population. Cataract as a cause of blindness appears in the fifth decade of life in southern Asia, whereas it appears in the sixth or seventh decade in most industrialized countries. A contributing factor to the high prevalence of blindness due to cataract in the developing world is the lack of an effective eye care delivery system.

Blindness registries are almost always incomplete, but in certain countries such registries may give some idea of the relative importance of the different causes of blindness. The *model reporting area* for blindness statistics in the USA revealed that cataract accounted for 12% of blindness.

The *number of operations for cataract* (cataract surgical rate) may provide a rough measure of the need for medical care that would be generated by cataracts in a particular population, but this rate is influenced by a number of factors, such as the availability of service, the visual requirements of the population in question, and the willingness of patients to undergo surgery. Moreover, surgical rates reflect only the number of operations performed and so do not represent the actual number of individuals with cataract or who may eventually have bilateral surgery. Although the annual cataract surgical rate is not available for most developing countries, data have been reported in industrialized countries. Rates vary from 100 to 5000 per 1 000 000 population in least developed and developed countries respectively.

Risk factors in cataract formation

Some studies suggest that lens opacities progress more rapidly in diabetics and that this progression occurs faster in diabetic women than in men. Another suspected risk factor, ultraviolet light or sunlight, has long been felt to contribute to cataract formation. This may be particularly significant in areas with high UVB irradiance levels. X-rays are known to induce cataracts in humans. Oral and topical corticosteroids and certain other drugs also produce cataract. It is possible that undernutrition and severe dehydrational states favour the development of cataract at an earlier age.

Methods of intervention

The diagnosis of clinically significant cataract is well defined and can be carried out by health personnel with minimal training. The larger problem is that of case-finding. The development of an efficient cataract surgery programme requires sample surveys to determine the magnitude of the problem, strategies for identifying and attracting cases to either a hospital or mobile eye unit and information concerning who will benefit from surgery. It is important to understand the social and behavioural factors that influence an individual patient's utilization of cataract surgery programmes. Increased promotion of cataract surgery and better visual rehabilitation, for example through the use of intraocular lens implantation, could play an important role in encouraging a patient's acceptance of surgery. The methods of case-finding and recruitment, the flow of patients and the preoperative and postoperative care of patients can vary from one country to another and even from one region to another in the same country.

There is no drug treatment for cataract, but sight can be restored by the surgical removal of the opaque (cataractous) lens and the provision of corrective spectacles or other devices. Appropriate technology is available to manufacture cataract spectacles at low cost in areas where these are not already available at affordable prices. On the other hand, significantly better quality of visual and functional outcome could result from the successful implantation of an intraocular lens after cataract removal. While the operation of choice is an extracapsular cataract extraction with a posterior chamber intraocular lens, good results have been reported with selected anterior chamber intraocular lenses following an intra-capsular cataract extraction. Another innovation in present-day patient management is curtailing the hospitalization period following surgery. However, ambulatory or day surgery is generally more feasible in developed countries or in urban areas in developing regions. Outpatient treatment obviates the need for expensive hospital beds and their attendant costs and could increase surgical turnover. The use of intraocular lens implantation, especially in monocular cataract, facilitates a low-cost period of rehabilitation. The cost of intraocular lenses, which in the past was an impediment to such surgery, has been markedly reduced by their production by non-commercial concerns in developing countries.

Action at various levels

Primary level

The initial intervention usually takes place at the primary level, where locally available health care personnel, such as the village health worker or volunteer, can be trained to screen for visual acuity and identify patients whose acuities are less than a predetermined level, usually 3/60 or 6/60. Further examinations to detect cataract can be carried out at the primary level, or patients can be referred directly to the secondary level.

Secondary level

The usual source of secondary-level care in most developing countries is the local hospital, staffed by a general medical practitioner and medical auxiliaries who have been trained to assist the general practitioner. Occasionally an ophthalmologist may be available, or at least a surgeon or general medical officer who has received training in cataract surgery. Cataract surgery should be available at the secondary level, where it can be performed in local hospitals, satellite eye hospitals or mobile eye units. Selection of cases is carried out at this level, and those needing surgery are scheduled for operative treatment.

Tertiary level

Tertiary facilities are primarily oriented towards care of more complicated cases like congenital cataracts requiring general anaesthesia, cataracts accompanied by other diseases of the eye such as glaucoma or iritis or cataracts associated with systemic diseases like diabetes that may complicate preoperative and postoperative care. In addition, the tertiary hospital may have facilities for intraocular lens surgery and can serve as a base for the development of satellite hospitals and mobile eye units and for the provision of training and outreach surgical services. To ensure a successful outcome in such surgery, emphasis should be placed on adequate training, the provision of appropriate equipment and supplies and careful postoperative follow-up. In view of the limited availability of these prerequisites, posterior chamber intraocular lens implantation may not always be a suitable standard method of cataract surgery in the primary health care environment or in outreach surgical services in most developing countries, at least in the short term.

Organizational aspects

Planning and integration

Ophthalmologists well trained in cataract surgery can deliver eye care to patients attending local hospitals. Where the transportation infrastructure is well developed, this is an especially feasible approach when hospitals are located in smaller cities relatively close to rural areas. However, since most hospitals are located in large cities and the majority of people in the developing world live in rural areas, these urban hospitals are not always ideal for the delivery of eye care to the outlying rural population. An outreach programme which can be integrated with district hospitals that are more accessible to the rural population may therefore be necessary in the short term.

Under certain conditions, the establishment of rural eye hospitals may be appropriate. These could be either general hospitals that are equipped and staffed to perform eye surgery, or satellite eye hospitals specifically organized for the delivery of eye care in the rural setting. Such satellite hospitals would serve the purpose not only of taking care of the backlog of cataract cases, but also of keeping up with new cases as they occur. Complicated cases, or cases requiring specialized treatment, such as retinal detachment surgery or vitrectomy, could be sent to the referral hospital.

The mobile eye unit is a third approach to eye care delivery and can serve both rural and urban areas where a permanent infrastructure for eye care is inadequate. This "eye camp" approach has already been established in some countries and is working satisfactorily to deliver services at the peripheral level. It requires detailed advance planning and community participation. To enhance the quality of surgical outcome, it is desirable that the eye camp approach be gradually phased out and static facilities utilized for surgery instead. However, in remote areas that are difficult to access, eye camps may still be needed for the foreseeable future in some countries. In all situations, strict adherence to surgical norms (before, during and after surgery) should be ensured.

Training

The personnel required will vary according to the needs in each country and may include senior and junior ophthalmologists, residents-in-training, ophthalmic assistants, ophthalmic technicians, nurses and voluntary personnel. If enough ophthalmologists are available, they can perform cataract surgery. Where intraocular lens surgery is to be introduced, training programmes to impart the required skills should be organized. In countries where the number of ophthalmologists available to remove cataracts in remote and disadvantaged communities is insufficient, the identification and training of general practitioners or other surgeons to organize and perform cataract surgery may be desirable. In instances where ophthalmic assistants or general nurses have received extensive training in cataract surgery, they may perform the surgery under supervision.

Auxiliary personnel play an important role in cataract surgery delivery. They may include categories such as ophthalmic assistants who test vision, measure intraocular pressure, irrigate nasolacrimal sacs and assist at surgery; nurses who manage preoperative and postoperative patient care; and aides who take care of the routine activities in the hospital or mobile eye unit. Flexibility in addressing personnel needs and application of the concept of teamwork are of the greatest importance in increasing productivity.

Evaluation

A periodic review of progress in reducing the magnitude of the cataract problem is important. This is best accomplished by focusing not solely on the number of operations performed, but also on the number of unoperated cases that remain in the population as determined by sample surveys. Information on the number and location of remaining cases is necessary for the efficient management of any programme designed to eliminate blindness due to cataract.

The performance of activities at every level should be evaluated periodically to ensure that care is adequate. Evaluation should be carried out with reference to the goals and objectives set at the outset. Sample surveys of patients who have undergone surgery should be conducted at intervals to help assess the performance of the team as a whole. Besides measuring the number of sight restoration operations performed, an assessment needs to be made of the outcome of surgery both in visual terms and in terms of quality of life and patient satisfaction.

Ocular trauma

Present state of knowledge

Description

Ocular trauma is the cause of blindness in more than half a million people worldwide and of partial loss of sight in many more. Trauma is often the leading cause of unilateral loss of vision, particularly in developing countries. However, the prevalence of blindness due to ocular trauma and the nature of associated injury vary widely in different parts of the world. In industrialized countries, the main risks are industrial and automobile accidents; in developing countries, the majority of injuries are from agricultural practices and cottage industries. Eye injuries are particularly frequent in rapidly industrializing countries because the hazards of the workplace are not yet appreciated by workers or their supervisors. In recent years, the rapid development of the chemical industry has resulted in a higher incidence of injuries caused by chemicals.

Blindness may be due to the initial injury or to a secondary infection and sympathetic ophthalmia. Injury and infection are often exacerbated by a delay in proper management and inappropriate home medication. The eye condition invariably worsens, and complications appear when time is lost through applying home medication instead of initiating proper medical management.

Trauma as a cause of blindness figures prominently in the list of causes of blindness and visual disability in many parts of the world, and has been reported as 0.8% in Zambia, 1.3% in India, 2.1% in China and Mali, 5.6% in Uganda, 6.7% in Sri Lanka and 9.4% in Fiji. It is also one of the common causes of absence from work. Thus, ocular injuries both generate a need for costly medical care and result in a loss of productivity.

Epidemiology

The pattern of incidence and the type and severity of ocular trauma are highly variable and are directly related to the setting in which they occur, i.e. civil or military, industrial or agricultural, occupational or domestic.

Poor midwifery can lead to serious birth trauma to the eyes. In the first two decades of life, eye injuries are common and severe. Children can damage their eyes when playing with dangerous toys like sticks, fireworks and missiles (e.g. darts or arrows). Boys are more prone to eye injury because of greater participation in outdoor activities and aggressive games; between 3% and 7.5% of accidents involving the eyes and adnexa are sports accidents, which tend to be particularly severe in terms of final outcome.

Occupational injuries account for a large proportion of eye trauma. In agricultural workers, injuries due to farming practices, and particularly to small foreign bodies such as wheat spikes, rice husks or sugar-cane leaves, account for a significant proportion of eye injuries. Exposure to toxic chemicals, particularly liquid ammonia, causes injury to the eye in both agricultural and industrial settings. Furthermore, a worldwide increase in automobile accidents results in many ocular injuries caused by splinters from the windshield and contusions. In particular circumstances, acute and chronic damage to the eye can be caused by a variety of electromagnetic radiation, including infrared, ultraviolet and ionizing radiation.

The nature of occupational trauma to the eye varies by country and situation. In developing countries, activities such as carpentry, black-smithing, stone-crushing, chiselling and hammering, and chopping wood are responsible for many eye injuries. During wars, combat-related blast injuries to the eyes are common.

Methods of intervention

In view of the varied nature of ocular trauma and inequalities in the availability of eye care services in remote areas, only general guidelines on the methods of intervention can be given.

Principles of prevention and treatment

Management of ocular trauma as part of primary eye care forms an integral part of health services. Primary health workers and trained personnel at peripheral posts should be able to organize preventive measures, undertake the initial management of ocular emergencies and arrange appropriate referrals.

Improved services for maternal and child health care can prevent many cases of trauma during birth; social and health education can reduce blindness caused by dangerous toys and games; increased awareness of the danger of agricultural and industrial practices, and the provision of facilities for first-aid can help reduce the magnitude of ocular trauma.

Education for eye safety should be integrated into the school syllabus at all levels. Playgrounds and children's parks that do not pose eye hazards should be provided in schools and residential areas.

Films on industrial and non-industrial ocular injuries can be prepared and the mass media used to create awareness of the need to prevent accidents and protect eyes. Issues such as the use of seatbelts and the dangers of fireworks should be included in public education.

In addition to health personnel, schoolteachers, social workers, volunteers and senior-level students can be trained to disseminate information on the prevention of ocular injuries.

Occupational safety

The key to the prevention of accidents in factories is to improve the safety features of machines, provide adequate illumination of working areas, select workers with alertness and good vision and encourage the use of protective devices.

Machine design should give high priority to the safety of the operator. Strict scrutiny of each machine is imperative before it leaves the factory to ensure that safety features are in place. There should be periodic inspection and maintenance of safety features.

Good illumination makes work easier and safer. Recommendations for lighting standards in factories should be sufficient to provide for adequate lighting.

Every possible effort should be made to improve the handling and storage of chemical materials that are injurious to the eye, such as caustics and acids.

The best method to safeguard the worker against ocular trauma is the use of proper protective devices such as goggles and face masks.

Visual standards and job placement

It is imperative for prospective workers to have good enough eyesight to carry out their jobs without endangering themselves or others. Appropriate guidelines for visual standards for various factory jobs should be developed. These should distinguish jobs requiring high visual efficiency, jobs requiring moderate visual efficiency and jobs requiring low visual efficiency.

Pre-employment visual records should be obtained and periodic check-ups carried out to ensure the safety of workers. Workers should be informed of possible hazards in their work and how to minimize their risk and be instructed in the use of personal protective devices.

Rural industries

Ocular injuries in rural populations, though frequent, tend to be relatively minor and often heal without serious damage to vision. However, secondary infection too often leads to gross visual impairment and blindness for lack of simple and timely intervention. The use of individual protective devices should be popularized. Simple, inexpensive and safe mechanical methods should be developed and made available to reduce direct manual handling of materials and livestock that pose risks to the eyes. Workers should accept responsibility for observing safety regulations.

The availability of primary eye care to treat minor injuries and prevent secondary infections is the most important means of reducing blindness due to trauma in the rural sector.

Automobile accidents

To prevent ocular injuries in automobile accidents, adequate automobile inspection and safety codes, a strict procedure for the awarding of driving licences and rules for the use of safety devices need to be adopted and enforced. Improved use of, and technology for, seatbelts, laminated windscreens and airbags in cars should reduce the occurrence of eye injuries in traffic accidents.

Radiation hazards

The adverse effects on the eyes of infrared (on glassblowers, in particular), ultraviolet and gamma radiation and X-rays are well known. Since the Second World War, there has been an increased awareness of radiation hazards to the eyes.

The use of radioactive materials in industry has introduced new hazards to both the individual worker and the general population. The increasing use of laser devices in military, industrial and domestic settings also presents a hazard to the eyes, and special safety measures should be defined.

Mining injuries

There is a high incidence of blindness in the mining industry, particularly as a result of the use of explosives. The great majority of these accidents are preventable by proper safety measures and training of workers.

Domestic and consumer safety

Public information and education are needed to reduce unnecessary dangers to the eyes, such as unsuitable packaging of potentially dangerous substances. Clear instructions should be provided on household products such as washing powders, solvents and paints as to what to do in case of contact with the eyes. Furthermore, in order to avoid domestic eye injuries in children, dangerous household products should be stored and used well out of their reach.

Action at various levels

Primary level

The treatment and management of ocular injuries are important parts of primary eye care in both rural and urban settings. Basic supplies of drugs, instruments and dressing materials should be provided to manage eye injuries at the primary level. It is of particular importance that antibiotic ointment be made available in rural areas.

The primary health care worker may remove *conjunctival* foreign bodies, but deeply embedded *corneal* foreign bodies are best dealt with by personnel with special training. If referral to the secondary or tertiary level is not practicable because of distance or for other reasons, it may be desirable to train primary health care workers in the removal of corneal foreign bodies, and to provide instruments, topical anaesthetics, antibiotic eye ointment and dressing material.

Each industry should make provision for first aid as well as for proper referral facilities for specialized care. Plants that pose serious risk because of chemical hazards should be assessed so that an emergency eye care service can be developed that emphasizes prevention and provides for quick irrigation and flushing of injurious toxic substances from the eyes. Periodic demonstrations using dummies can be effective.

Secondary and tertiary levels

In addition to emergency measures that can be applied on-site, some patients will need further treatment at the district hospital or more specialized treatment in tertiary centres. Information regarding the eye injury service should be readily available and liaison with secondary and tertiary hospital authorities should be maintained.

Organizational aspects

Planning and integration

Prevention of injuries is a matter of great public health significance. Coordinating action by governmental and other agencies in the area of eye safety should be promoted through school committees (consisting of teachers, students, parents and a health worker), village committees (local leaders and health workers), and industrial committees (employer, workers, industrial and safety engineers and a health worker). Eye safety guidelines and trauma reporting and surveillance should be established by these committees.

All efforts should include the dissemination of safety guidelines and recommendations on how to prevent ocular injury within the community. Managers of industry must ensure that essential first-aid measures are provided and that a record is kept of potential causes of ocular injury.

Legislation should be promoted to:

— prohibit the use of untrained labour in high-risk jobs;
— enforce minimum safety standards for workshops and factories with regard to lighting and the maximum number of working hours;
— regulate the manufacture and use of fireworks;
— make mandatory the provision and use of protective devices in high-risk areas;
— make mandatory the provision of first-aid equipment and kits in high-risk industries;
— make mandatory the availability and use of seatbelts in cars;
— make mandatory the safe packaging and distribution to the consumer of dangerous chemicals and other substances.

Evaluation

The outcome of interventions and treatment requires evaluation. Several standard forms are in use for these purposes. A standard international reporting form would be useful, covering such areas as the cause and severity of injury, the extent of initial damage due to trauma, the presence of secondary infection and the extent of ultimate damage.

Training

Prevention of ocular trauma necessarily involves the training in safe practices of those who design, use and maintain machines. Close contact between medical and engineering personnel is therefore imperative.

Engineers in specific industries should receive short training courses on ocular hazards and how to prevent ocular injury.

Training and refresher courses should be organized for factory managers, engineers, factory doctors and eye specialists to inform them of the latest advances in the field of prevention and management of eye trauma.

Science teachers in schools and colleges should be trained in safety precautions and first aid. Basic health workers need to be adequately trained in the relevant aspects of ocular trauma, with stress on prevention and first aid. Medical staff at the peripheral level and those associated with industry and emergency rooms should attend regular refresher courses on the epidemiology of ocular injuries, their prevention and their treatment.

People working in hazardous occupations should have adequate practical training in their jobs before they operate machines or handle chemicals; the value of protective eye-wear should be explained and its use made mandatory. Employees should be trained in simple first-aid measures by experienced personnel; the training should be practical and should be repeated periodically.

At the tertiary level, training should inculcate the necessary expertise to deal with ocular trauma and its complications.

Glaucoma

Present state of knowledge

Description

The understanding of glaucoma has changed in the past decade as a result of new epidemiological information, improved diagnostic methods and developments in surgical and drug therapy.

Glaucoma includes four distinct entities, with the common but not obligatory feature of intraocular pressure high enough to impair the functioning of the optic nerve and cause visual field loss ultimately leading to blindness. The four disease entities are: congenital or infantile glaucoma, primary open-angle glaucoma, primary angle-closure glaucoma and secondary glaucoma.

Glaucoma remains an important cause of blindness, both in developing and in industrialized countries. It accounts for approximately 15% of all blindness. It has been estimated that about 5 200 000 persons have been rendered blind from glaucoma (3 000 000 from primary open-angle glaucoma; 2 000 000 from primary angle-closure glaucoma; 200 000 from congenital or infantile glaucoma). Glaucoma is responsible for approximately 600 000 new cases of blindness per year worldwide.

Primary open-angle glaucoma and primary angle-closure glaucoma account for the vast majority of cases of glaucoma-related blindness. Of the two, primary open-angle glaucoma is more common and also more difficult to diagnose and treat. In developing countries, with a large backlog of unoperated hypermature cataracts, lens-induced secondary glaucoma adds to the magnitude of the problem.

Primary open-angle glaucoma is a slowly progressing, insidious eye disease, which is difficult to detect because it is nearly asymptomatic. It usually affects both eyes. A particular appearance of the optic disc (head of the optic nerve) and a slowly progressive loss of visual sensitivity are the classic signs.

The typical characteristic of the glaucomatous optic disc (i.e. excavation) is visible by ophthalmoscopy, and the present standard for determining visual loss is the visual field test. In patients with primary open-angle glaucoma there is usually also an elevation of intraocular pressure. However, elevated intraocular pressure is no longer part of the definition of the disease, since many glaucoma patients have intraocular pressure that falls within the normal range.

Intraocular pressure is usually elevated for many years before the onset of characteristic field loss, although patients with higher pressures tend to develop loss of visual field sooner. Because intraocular pressure rises slowly and central vision is retained until late, the patient usually remains unaware of the problem until it is too late for effective treatment.

In spite of notable advances, the recognition and treatment of primary open-angle glaucoma are still unsatisfactory, even in industrialized countries.

Epidemiological studies have made an important contribution by determining some of the essential risk factors for glaucoma and some of the criteria for identification of people with suspected primary open-angle glaucoma. Thus:

— high intraocular pressure is the most consistent risk factor (which is why the definition of primary open-angle glaucoma used to include a minimal pressure level);

— older age is consistently found to predispose patients to eye damage (the prevalence of primary open-angle glaucoma increases rapidly after the age of 40 years);

— race has been consistently reported as an important risk factor (black populations have a rate of glaucoma four to eight times higher than that of Caucasian populations);

— kinship with a patient with primary open-angle glaucoma is also a risk factor (the genetic basis of primary open-angle glaucoma is currently under intense study);

— high blood pressure, diabetes and myopia have been implicated as risk factors in some reports (there is still conflicting evidence regarding the possible association between primary open-angle glaucoma and alcohol intake or smoking).

Primary angle-closure glaucoma is a rarer condition among Caucasians than primary open-angle glaucoma (accounting for about 10% of glaucoma in this population) but is more common among Asians. Progress has been made in epidemiology and screening in high-risk subpopulations, notably Inuit people, but much remains to be done in the larger populations of Asia where the condition is more frequently diagnosed.

This condition occurs when the intraocular pressure rises rapidly due to the sudden blockage of the trabecular meshwork by the iris root. The attack may be facilitated by pupil dilation, whether physiological or pharmacological. It is manifested by pain, blurred vision (the rise of intraocular pressure causes corneal oedema which is responsible for the visual symptoms), rainbow-coloured halos around lights, nausea and vomiting.

Signs of acute primary angle-closure glaucoma include high intraocular pressure, a mid-dilated, non-reactive and often irregular pupil, corneal oedema, a shallow anterior chamber and congested conjunctival blood vessels around the cornea.

During an acute attack, intraocular pressure may be high enough to cause glaucomatous optic nerve damage or retinal vascular occlusion, leading to irreversible ocular damage and ultimately blindness, usually within 1–3 days. Primary angle-closure glaucoma is an ocular emergency and must be referred and treated properly for vision to be preserved.

In general, primary angle-closure glaucoma is a bilateral disease: an untreated fellow eye has a 40–80% chance of developing an acute attack within 5–10 years. For this reason, it is routine to operate on both eyes, rather than only on the eye that presents the acute attack.

Congenital and infantile glaucoma. Primary infantile glaucoma accounts for about one-half of childhood glaucomas, the rest being associated with other ocular and congenital conditions. Infantile glaucoma is a rare disorder. Sixty per cent of cases are diagnosed by the age of 6 months. (The term congenital glaucoma should be reserved for those cases with signs of glaucoma present at birth.) Elevated intraocular pressure during the first years of life results in optic atrophy and often enlargement of the eyeball and cloudiness of the cornea. The natural history of this disorder is devastating, and management requires specialized surgery.

Secondary glaucomas are caused by a large number of ocular diseases. Prevention depends on the prevention or treatment of the underlying disease.

Diagnosis

Patients developing primary open-angle glaucoma are generally asymptomatic. Diagnosis can be made with certainty if facilities are available for the measurement of intraocular pressure, examination of the optic disc and testing of the visual fields. To make the diagnosis, the ophthalmologist notes the history to establish known risk factors and performs an examination including tonometry, ophthalmoscopy, gonioscopy (to examine the angle of the anterior chamber) and visual field testing.

The standard instrument for measuring intraocular pressure is Goldmann's aplanation tonometer, typically used with the slit-lamp (other tonometers include Schiotz and non-contact devices). Special screening procedures using mainly tonometry are often carried out on apparently healthy adults (over 30–40 years of age) in order to identify early cases. Unfortunately, there is no satisfactory threshold pressure in screening for primary open-angle glaucoma. A pressure value of 21 mmHg (2.8 kPa) has a sensitivity of 65% and a specificity of 91.7%. The accuracy and reliability of tonometry are affected to some extent by the choice of device, the experience of the examiner and physiological variables in the patient. A single measurement of intraocular pressure has limited negative predictive value in ruling out glaucoma. No single value provides a reasonable balance of sensitivity and specificity. Furthermore, the ability of eyes to withstand elevated intraocular pressure varies widely and, unless the pressure is consistently very high, it is impossible to predict how soon, or whether, a given eye will develop characteristic field loss.

The optic disc can be examined to identify the excavation typical of glaucoma and to estimate the cup-to-disc ratio. Unfortunately, unless the optic disc is actually seen to enlarge over time, to be very large to begin with or to be asymmetric in comparison with the fellow eye, it is impossible to be certain from disc appearance alone that the patient has primary open-angle glaucoma, since many individuals have large optic cups. Nevertheless, the association of elevated intraocular pressure and large optic cups (or different-sized cups in the two eyes) would strongly suggest primary open-angle glaucoma. Gonioscopy as performed during a slit-lamp examination, with a hand-held lens, allows for assessment of the chamber angle.

The definitive diagnosis of primary open-angle glaucoma requires a finding of decreased visual function on testing with a visual field instrument. Today, automated systems are more sensitive for the detection of glaucomatous scotoma than previous manual procedures. Visual field testing—although clearly of vital importance in screening since other methods lack adequate sensitivity—is time-consuming, requires a high degree of cooperation and is subject to many sources of error (lack of standardization, etc.). It is therefore usually not feasible in large-scale interventions in developing countries.

There is now great interest in developing "new" tests of visual function that would allow the diagnosis of glaucoma before the onset of visual field loss (e.g. contrast sensitivity, acuity perimetry, visual evoked response).

Screening effectively for glaucoma is difficult. It is not uncommon to use two-stage screening techniques: large populations are examined for elevated pressures and individuals found to have high pressures are referred for visual field examination. However, only one out of every 30 people thus referred will actually have a glaucomatous field loss and one-third to one-half of those with field loss will have had a normal intraocular pressure when screened. Screening procedures are thus inefficient and not cost-effective.

In comparison with primary open-angle glaucoma, the diagnosis of primary angle-closure glaucoma is clinically easier. The condition is diagnosed by the presence of pain, visual loss, a red eye, a large, non-reactive pupil, a cloudy cornea, indicative gonioscopy findings and elevated pressure in an eye with a shallow anterior chamber.

Methods of intervention

Because there are several distinct disease processes, there is no single method for the prevention of visual loss by "glaucoma".

Primary open-angle glaucoma cannot be prevented. Its treatment is still controversial. Since high intraocular pressure is a major risk factor, it is logical that reducing pressure could have therapeutic benefit. Drugs such as pilocarpine, epinephrine and β-adrenergic blockers are used to lower pressure and to prevent visual loss from progressive destruction of the optic nerve fibres. The protective effect is not absolute.

If medical therapy is ineffective, those at high risk are selected for surgical pressure-lowering treatment: laser and/or incisional therapy (filtering procedures). Unfortunately, traditional surgery is probably the only means of therapy applicable to developing countries, where the cost of drugs is prohibitive, the close follow-up required for effective adjustment of drug therapy is inapplicable and lasers are unavailable.

Primary angle-closure glaucoma is a medical emergency requiring prompt reduction in intraocular pressure and removal of the blockage of flow between the posterior and anterior chambers. Patients should receive an oral hyperosmotic agent, such as glycerol, and frequent topical miotics (e.g. pilocarpine 4%) until the angle is open. As soon as the eye is white and pain-free, and the pressure normal, a peripheral iridectomy should be performed to prevent future attacks. To forestall an attack in the other eye, the patient should receive pilocarpine 1% twice a day until a peripheral iridectomy can be performed.

Where a laser is available, a laser iridotomy can be performed as an outpatient procedure. Otherwise, a surgical peripheral iridectomy should be done in the affected eye as well as in the fellow eye. After an iridectomy or iridotomy, patients should be examined periodically for as long as they remain available for follow-up.

Action at various levels

Primary level

All primary health care workers should be able to recognize that an acute red eye with reduced vision, pain, corneal clouding or a dilated pupil requires immediate referral to rule out, or treat, angle-closure glaucoma.

There is little the primary health care worker can do to identify patients with early open-angle glaucoma. He or she should recognize the need, however, to refer patients with decreased visual acuity, particularly when the problem is unilateral, as well as patients with relatively fixed, dilated or asymmetric pupils.

There is insufficient rationale to recommend the routine performance of tonometry by primary care physicians as a screening test for glaucoma. It may be clinically prudent, however, to advise patients at high risk (those aged 65 years and more, black people or close relatives of a glaucoma patient) to be tested periodically for glaucoma by an eye specialist or trained ophthalmic clinical officer.

Secondary level

Personnel at the secondary level should be capable of differentiating between the various causes of red eye and providing appropriate medical therapy. Whenever possible, they should have available both pilocarpine and oral hyperosmotic agents such as glycerol to treat angle closure. Depending upon their degree of training in ophthalmic disease, secondary-level personnel may perform peripheral iridectomies. Otherwise these operations should be performed at the tertiary level.

For chronic open-angle glaucoma, the challenge at the secondary level is case-detection. Patients with possible disease should be referred to the tertiary level for evaluation and filtering surgery if needed. Following successful surgery, the patient should return to the secondary-level worker for periodic evaluation and re-referral if intraocular pressure begins to rise again.

Tertiary level

Depending upon the quality and relative availability of services at the secondary and tertiary levels, tertiary-level personnel may be required to perform peripheral iridectomies. Because of their superior training and facilities, they are best equipped to carry out filtering surgery and surgical-laser therapy, and to manage early postoperative complications.

Certain diagnostic procedures (tonometry, perimetry) may be delegated to appropriately trained and supervised personnel. However, the final interpretation of the results and the responsibility for management of glaucoma require the experience and expertise of an ophthalmologist.

Before the development of effective surgical therapy, infantile glaucoma almost always resulted in blindness. As medications appear to have a limited long-term value, the preferred therapy is surgical. Infants with suspected disease need prompt referral to a tertiary-level eye institution.

Organizational aspects

Training

Primary eye care workers should receive instruction in the recognition of, and need for, immediate referral of patients with red eyes and pain or decreased vision.

At the very least, personnel at the secondary level should be trained to diagnose and manage acute angle-closure glaucoma. They should also be trained to perform tonometry, to examine the optic disc and visual fields and to diagnose chronic open-angle glaucoma. In some instances they may be trained to perform peripheral iridectomies.

Personnel at the tertiary level should receive adequate training to examine the anterior chamber angle (gonioscopy) and to manage chronic open-angle glaucoma medically and surgically and congenital glaucoma surgically.

Screening

Screening the entire population for glaucoma has not been found to be cost-effective. However, screening individuals or groups at high risk is considerably more efficient.

Availability of drugs

To control glaucoma, the availability of eye drops is essential.

In general, a drug shortage is experienced mostly at the primary level and in remote areas. This issue can be considered from several points of view:

— the range of preparations available;
— the supply (regular or not);
— the shelf-life and effective delivery date at each level of health care;
— the affordability (for the health system or the patient).

Emphasis should be placed by national health authorities on ensuring that an adequate range of glaucoma medicine is regularly available at the primary level. It will consequently be necessary to identify affordable preparations and to track them through the various stages of delivery in order to allow for a useful shelf-life when the medications are made accessible to the patient.

Diabetic retinopathy

Present state of knowledge

Description

Diabetic retinopathy is the leading cause of blindness in working-age people. Although diabetes mellitus has been predominantly a disease of developed countries, its incidence is increasing in less developed countries as well. It now displays a single epidemiological profile worldwide.

Diabetic retinopathy is characterized by microaneurysm formation (localized dilation of capillaries) and the presence of small haemorrhages such that the retina shows scattered red dots. These changes constitute *background diabetic retinopathy*. Progressive leakage from capillaries and microaneurysms results in the retinal swelling and decreased vision known as macular oedema, which is the most important cause of blindness in diabetic retinopathy. *Proliferative diabetic retinopathy* is characterized by new blood vessel growth, either at the disc (neovascularization of the disc) or elsewhere (neovascularization elsewhere). Rupture of these vessels creates blinding vitreous haemorrhage, and progressive scar tissue formation following this "scaffolding" of new blood vessels causes traction retinal detachment.

Laser photocoagulation reduces the risk of blindness by more than 60% and possibly by as much as 95%. However, it must be carried out before vision deteriorates, and patients must be followed very closely.

Lost vision cannot be regained. Laser treatment works best to *prevent* visual loss—hence, patients must be identified *before* overt symptoms develop, either by regular community screening or through individual self-referral for eye examination.

Epidemiology

Diabetic eye disease is an increasingly important cause of blindness in developing countries as diabetes mellitus increases in prevalence and other causes of blindness are better managed. Work throughout the islands of the South Pacific, for instance, has highlighted the increasing incidence of diabetes mellitus as a more urban lifestyle is adopted. The trends throughout these communities show that similar risk factors are operative worldwide and that the duration of diabetes is the most important predictor for the development of diabetic retinopathy.

Some degree of diabetic retinopathy develops in virtually all diabetics after 20 years. Once diabetic retinopathy is present, sight-threatening retinopathy develops in 6% of patients per year:

— 4% with macular oedema;
— 2% with proliferative diabetic retinopathy.

Diagnosis

Diabetic retinopathy is characterized by microaneurysms and micro-haemorrhages; both appear as small red dots in the retina. Oedematous residues from macular oedema show as yellowish dots or streaks, whereas neovascularization is seen as irregularly arranged preretinal vessels with sausage-like venous dilation and nerve-fibre infarcts (whitish-grey "cotton wool" spots near the optic nerve). Vitreous haemorrhage forms showers of small red dots or obscures the fundal view.

Diabetic retinopathy is best assessed by a trained observer looking through the dilated pupil with a slit-lamp or at retinal photographs. A direct ophthalmoscope will allow detection of background and proliferative retinopathy but not evaluation of macular oedema. All specifically trained eye health workers should be able to detect diabetic retinopathy and refer patients to a treatment centre.

Methods of intervention

Since laser treatment must be carried out before visual acuity deteriorates, the detection of potentially blinding complications by examining asymptomatic diabetics is essential. This can be achieved either through a mass screening programme, where people present themselves once a year for an eye examination or for retinal photographs, or by means of an individual visiting an eye care provider. Both clinical examination by an experienced observer and photography have similar detection rates, so the choice of method should be guided by the personnel and financial resources available in the local community.

Assessment of the severity of retinopathy requires a retinal examination through a dilated pupil, in order to provide stereoscopic evaluation of retinal thickness and to make possible detailed examination of the mid-peripheral retina for neovascularization. Retinopathy cannot be adequately assessed using a direct ophthalmoscope and certainly cannot be assessed by the patient's clarity of sight. Standard diagnostic methods include slit-lamp biomicroscopy of the retina, colour photography and, in selected cases, fluorescein angiography.

Fluorescein angiography involves the injection of sodium fluorescein into the antecubital vein during sequential photography. Sodium fluorescein has several crucial features: it is a non-toxic small molecule that stays within normal retinal vessels but leaks out of abnormal vessels into areas of macular oedema. Fluorescein angiography is used to establish the fine diagnostic features of retinopathy and to guide treatment. The possible side-effects include nausea, vomiting (in fewer than 5% of cases) and, very rarely, anaphylaxis.

The cornerstone of retinopathy treatment is early laser photo-coagulation, which is indicated for proliferative retinopathy and macular oedema. Laser treatment is an outpatient procedure in which the patient sits with his or her head supported on a chin-and-forehead rest and the retina is viewed through a special contact lens. A fine laser beam (commonly 0.2 mm in diameter) is used either to ablate the peripheral retina for proliferative disease or to cauterize leaking dilated capillaries locally. Generally, this is performed with topical anaesthesia (drops), although occasionally treatment is uncomfortable and a retrobulbar injection of a local anaesthetic (lidocaine) is necessary. After treatment, the vision is often dull for a period. The eye is patched for between 30 minutes and 6 hours, depending on the type of anaesthetic used. Patients may go home immediately and are advised to avoid straining their vision. Rarely, a corneal abrasion develops that will heal within 12 hours if the eye is firmly patched. Patients can be reassured that laser treatment does not involve hospitalization or the risks of general anaesthesia.

Vitrectomy is a major ocular operation reserved for vitreous haemorrhage or traction retinal detachment. As it is a microsurgical procedure there is often little pain or discomfort, and it can be performed under local or general anaesthesia. Patients are generally in hospital for several days. Major blinding complications can occur after vitrectomy, and it is carried out only in selected centres where expensive microscopes and vitrectomy instrumentation are available. Vision may be reduced for weeks afterwards.

Other forms of treatment (e.g. drugs) have a limited role. Aspirin has been shown to have no positive or negative influence on the progression of diabetic retinopathy. Somatostatin analogues and aldose reductase inhibitors are being studied but these therapies are in an investigational phase only. The discarded therapy of pituitary ablation has no place in diabetic management.

Action at various levels

Primary level

The prevention of diabetes, if possible, is the ideal. Attention should be focused on changes in lifestyle to reduce the risk of diabetes. Moreover, strict control of blood-sugar levels reduces the risk of severe complications in a diabetes patient.

Secondary level

All health workers should be trained to recognize the symptoms and signs of diabetes. People with non-insulin dependent diabetes should be examined for diabetic retinopathy, including clinically significant macular oedema and proliferative disease, at the time of initial diagnosis. If no retinopathy is present, it is generally safe to wait 5 years before further ocular examination. Once diabetic retinopathy is detected, review should be yearly or more frequent depending on the severity of retinopathy. Insulin-dependent diabetics should be examined 5 years after onset of the condition and yearly thereafter.

A pregnant woman with pre-existing diabetes runs the risk of rapid progression of diabetic retinopathy. She should have a detailed ophthalmoscopic examination early in pregnancy and follow-up during the course of pregnancy.

Laser treatment should be performed when high-risk characteristics are detected—either clinically significant macular oedema or neovascularization of the disc or elsewhere.

Tertiary level

The development of vitreous haemorrhage or traction retinal detachment requires referral to a tertiary management centre where intraocular microsurgery can be performed. This is a highly skilled procedure requiring expensive equipment and is restricted to a small number of specialized centres. Depending on the financial realities of the community involved, transfer to a competent centre should be considered.

Organizational aspects

Primary eye care workers should be trained to understand the characteristics of diabetic retinopathy and the importance of regular screening to detect its early stages. Personnel at the secondary level should have received adequate instruction to diagnose clinically significant macular oedema or proliferative retinopathy and arrange appropriate laser treatment either locally or at a treatment centre. Physicians, general practitioners and other health personnel who examine or treat patients with diabetes should be made aware of the sight-threatening nature of diabetic retinopathy and of the need for periodic eye examination through referral. Tertiary-level care of diabetic retinopathy is not feasible for many communities because of the high cost of equipment and training of personnel. However, the establishment of regional specialist centres should be encouraged.

Childhood blindness

Present state of knowledge

General aspects and epidemiology

Prevalence

There are few sources of population-based data on the prevalence of childhood blindness and low vision and no sources of data on their incidence. In industrialized countries, some information is available from blindness registries, and population-based studies of adult blindness in developing countries have given some crude estimates of the prevalence of blindness in children. In general terms, the prevalence of childhood blindness is at least three to five times greater in poor areas of the world than in industrialized countries. It is estimated that there are approximately 1.5 million blind children in the world (Table 7), and an estimated 500000 become blind each year, of whom probably more than half die in childhood. The prevalence of low vision is probably three to four times greater than that of blindness, with approximately 5 million children being affected worldwide.

Causes

There are two distinct ways of classifying causes of childhood blindness and low vision. The first is a descriptive, anatomical classification according to the level at which vision is obstructed in the eye (Table 8).

The second classification is by etiology, according to the developmental time at which the insult occurred (Table 9).

It is usually easier to describe the cause of visual loss anatomically than etiologically, but both classifications are important in the management and treatment of individual children and can be used for identifying and monitoring preventive strategies.

Most of the information on the causes of childhood blindness and low vision has come from the examination of children in schools for the blind.

Table 7. Estimated magnitude of childhood blindness by region

Region	Population < 16 years of age (millions)	Blindness prevalence (per 1000 children)	Estimated number of blind children
Africa	240	1.1	264000
Asia	1200	0.9	1080000
Central and South America	130	0.6	78000
Europe/Japan/USA	240	0.3	72000
TOTAL	1810		1494000

Table 8. Anatomical classification of causes of childhood blindness and low vision

Whole globe	e.g. microphthalmos, anophthalmos, phthisis bulbi
Cornea	e.g. corneal scarring, anterior staphyloma, dystrophies
Lens	e.g. cataract, dislocated lens
Uvea	e.g. aniridia, chronic uveitis, coloboma
Retina	e.g. retinopathy of prematurity, retinal dystrophies, retinal detachment
Glaucoma	e.g. buphthalmos
Optic nerve	e.g. optic atrophy, optic nerve hypoplasia
Other	e.g. cortical blindness, amblyopia

Table 9. Etiological classification of childhood blindness and low vision

Hereditary	e.g. autosomal dominant or recessive disease, chromosomal abnormalities
Intrauterine	e.g. congenitally acquired rubella, fetal alcohol syndrome
Perinatal	e.g. ophthalmia neonatorum, retinopathy of prematurity
Childhood	e.g. vitamin A deficiency, measles, harmful traditional eye practices, trauma
Unclassified	e.g. impossible to determine the underlying cause

For various reasons, these results may not be representative of the total population of visually impaired children, as the schools tend to be in cities and usually admit children from older age groups, so that preschool children, children from rural areas and also those with additional disabilities may not be adequately represented.

The main causes of childhood blindness in developing countries are preventable and include conditions that give rise to corneal scarring, e.g. vitamin A deficiency, measles, harmful traditional eye practices, ophthalmia neonatorum and other corneal infections. Potentially treatable conditions include cataract and glaucoma.

In industrialized countries, the main causes of childhood visual loss are lesions of the central nervous system and hereditary diseases (particularly affecting the retina), some of which may be amenable to preventive measures such as genetic counselling. Retinopathy of prematurity, which is a potentially avoidable cause of childhood blindness, is important where very-low-birth-weight babies (less than 1500 g) survive. Congenital cataract and congenital glaucoma together represent 10–20% of childhood blindness in most parts of the world.

Methods of intervention

In most regions of the world, approximately 50% of children in schools for the blind have blindness that could have been prevented (Table 10).

The optimal control strategies and methods of intervention will depend on the causes of blindness and low vision in the country concerned. Before

Table 10. Avoidable causes of childhood blindness: from studies in schools for the blind

Region	Preventable conditions	(%)	Treatable conditions	(%)	% avoidable
West Africa	VAD/measles/TEP ON Rubella	39	Glaucoma Cataract Others	31	70
Southern India	VAD ADH disease ON	37	Cataract Glaucoma Others	10	47
Thailand/ Philippines	VAD ON Rubella	33	ROP Cataract Glaucoma	26	59
Chile	ADH disease Rubella ON	18	ROP Cataract Glaucoma	36	54

Abbreviations: VAD = vitamin A deficiency
TEP = harmful traditional eye practices
ON = ophthalmia neonatorum
ROP = retinopathy of prematurity
ADH = autosomal dominant hereditary (disease)

planning what services to offer, it is important to identify the major preventable and treatable conditions, so that resources can be allocated to the most "controllable" and prevalent conditions which cause the most preventable morbidity. This can be done by examining children in schools for the blind and by collecting data from hospital clinics or blindness registries. A form has been developed for recording the causes of blindness and low vision in children that allows for the collection of data in a standardized manner.[1]

Action at various levels

Primary level

Vitamin A deficiency and measles

In regions of the world where corneal scarring is the main cause of childhood blindness, children should be examined for signs of night blindness or Bitot's spots, which are likely to be caused by vitamin A deficiency and can lead to corneal ulceration and blindness. All children with signs of xerophthalmia should be treated with vitamin A (for treatment schedule, see Table 3). Vitamin A should also be given to any child with a measles infection, obvious malnutrition or diarrhoea of more than 1 week's duration. Communities of children with levels of xerophthalmia that indicate vitamin A deficiency is a public health problem should be targeted with measures that promote vitamin A intake as well as measles immunization, nutritional education, diarrhoea control and vitamin A supplementation (for recommended schedules, see Table 4).

Eye infections

Prophylaxis against ophthalmia neonatorum—cleansing the eyes of newborn babies immediately after delivery (before the eyes open) and applying tetracycline 1% eye ointment (or 1 drop of silver nitrate 1% solution)—will prevent conjunctivitis in the newborn and the danger of gonococcal corneal ulceration.

Treatment of conjunctivitis in children with antibiotic eye ointment is an important element of eye care at the primary level, as is health education regarding the use of harmful traditional eye practices.

---

[1] Gilbert C et al. Childhood blindness: a new form for recording causes of visual loss in children. *Bulletin of the World Health Organization*, 1993, 71(5):485–489.

Immunization

As well as measles immunization, rubella immunization may be indicated in all 1-year-old children and in girls aged 10–12 years. Prevention of congenitally acquired rubella, which can cause cataract, glaucoma or microphthalmos, is the major objective of vaccinating girls before puberty.

Secondary level

The management of ocular injuries and corneal ulcers in children is undertaken at the secondary level by trained health workers and ophthalmologists.

The provision of spectacles for children with refractive errors is carried out by ophthalmologists, ophthalmic assistants and optometrists. Children with a visual loss that is not correctable by refraction (e.g. amblyopia) and those with ocular abnormalities are likely to need referral for examination and treatment at the tertiary level.

Tertiary level

Retinopathy of prematurity

Very-low-birth-weight babies (below 1500 g) and those born at less than 32 weeks' gestation require examination to identify retinopathy of prematurity needing treatment, i.e. "stage 3" or more advanced disease.[1] Examination should be by indirect ophthalmoscopy, and the first examination should be performed 6–7 weeks after birth, with further examinations at intervals of 1–2 weeks if indicated. Stage 3 or more advanced disease is an indication for cryotherapy or laser photocoagulation to reduce the incidence of visually disabling complications.

Surgically treatable eye conditions of childhood

For the surgical treatment of childhood cataract, glaucoma, retinopathy of prematurity and strabismus, only tertiary centres are likely to be able to provide the surgical expertise and long-term follow-up required to obtain good visual results.

Spectacles and refractive devices

Spectacles and refractive devices are extremely important to maximize the visual potential of children with an impairment. This requires assessment,

---

[1] *Prevention of childhood blindness.* Geneva, World Health Organization, 1992:14.

the use of appropriate optical devices and magnifiers, and motivation by a low-vision therapist on how to use the devices. Such a service, whether for children in schools for the visually impaired or in integrated education, is likely to be coordinated from the tertiary centre.

Screening

Screening at birth

All children should, if possible, have an external examination of the eyes at, or shortly after, birth. A simple examination with a torch is sufficient to detect the following conditions:

— *buphthalmos*: a large eye or eyes, often with a hazy cornea due to congenital glaucoma;
— *leukocoria*: a white pupil from congenital cataract, retinoblastoma or other congenital anomalies;
— *ophthalmia neonatorum*: a purulent discharge from the eye or eyes;
— obvious abnormalities: anophthalmos (missing eye); microphthalmos (small eye).

If any of these abnormalities is detected the child should be referred for detailed ocular examination and treatment.

Parents may notice that their baby has an ocular abnormality, fails to look at or follow an object or develops rapid involuntary ocular movements (nystagmus). These observations should be taken seriously and the child referred for ocular examination. In case of doubt, and if facilities exist, electro-diagnostic tests may be indicated to determine whether the retina and optic nerve are functioning normally.

Preschool screening

Where feasible, preschool screening helps identify children with squints (strabismus) and possibly also amblyopia. Early treatment could be instituted to prevent irreversible visual loss.

School screening

Screening of schoolchildren for visual loss can be performed by trained health workers or schoolteachers. Children with a visual acuity of 6/12 or less in either eye should be referred for refraction and ophthalmic examination. The commonest causes of visual loss at this age are refractive errors (for which spectacles may be indicated) and amblyopia.

In areas with endemic vitamin A deficiency or trachoma, affected schoolchildren should be identified and treated. The school population also offers an opportunity for health education about "healthy eyes".

Organizational aspects

Planning and integration

Control of childhood blindness at the primary level should be integrated into existing programmes and services, i.e. maternal and child health clinics, child survival programmes, the Expanded Programme on Immunization, well-baby clinics and community health services. In regions of the world where corneal scarring is a problem, adequate supplies of vitamin A and topical antibiotics, such as tetracycline eye ointment, should be available. Immunization against measles is important, and the use of harmful traditional practices should be discouraged. At the secondary and tertiary levels, close cooperation between ophthalmologists and other health personnel involved in child health, such as neonatologists and paediatricians, is required. Special equipment for the examination and management of children with treatable disease is necessary at the secondary and tertiary levels.

Training

Because the causes of childhood blindness vary from region to region, it is not possible to provide detailed recommendations for training that would apply universally. The following are broad guidelines.

Primary level

Primary health workers should be trained so that they have sufficient knowledge for the following:

— to institute appropriate measures to prevent childhood blindness from ophthalmia neonatorum and vitamin A deficiency;
— to identify and manage conditions that need treatment, i.e. xerophthalmia, measles infection, conjunctivitis and trachoma;
— to recognize conditions that require referral to a higher centre, i.e. cataract, glaucoma, retinoblastoma, visual loss without obvious cause, strabismus and ocular injuries.

Selected groups of individuals like schoolteachers can be trained in visual acuity testing and given guidelines on referral.

Secondary level

Training at the secondary level includes the diagnosis and management of corneal ulceration and trauma and the identification of conditions requiring referral.

Tertiary level

There is a need to develop specialist, tertiary-level units where ophthalmologists are available who are trained in the management of conditions requiring a high level of expertise, such as congenital cataract and glaucoma, retinopathy of prematurity, etc.

Low-vision services with trained optometrists and low-vision therapists should also be developed.

Evaluation

The impact of specific interventions, such as vitamin A supplementation and measles immunization, can be evaluated by monitoring changes in the incidence of xerophthalmia and corneal scarring. The impact of other control measures can be monitored by recording changes in the pattern of childhood blindness over time through a register or surveys that record the causes of visual loss using the standardized methodology.

References and selected further reading

Trachoma

Dawson CR, Jones BR, Tarizzo ML. *Guide to trachoma control in programmes for the prevention of blindness.* Geneva, World Health Organization, 1981.

Reacher M, Foster A, Huber J. *Trichiasis surgery for trachoma: the bilamellar tarsal rotation procedure.* Geneva, World Health Organization, 1993 (unpublished document WHO/PBL/93.29; available on request from Programme for the Prevention of Blindness and Deafness, World Health Organization, 1211 Geneva 27, Switzerland).

Primary health care level management of trachoma. Geneva, World Health Organization, 1993 (unpublished document WHO/PBL/93.33; available on request from Programme for the Prevention of Blindness and Deafness, World Health Organization, 1211 Geneva 27, Switzerland).

Francis V, Turner V. *Achieving community support for trachoma control: a guide for district health work.* Geneva, World Health Organization, 1993 (unpublished document WHO/PBL/93.36; available on request from Programme for the Prevention of Blindness and Deafness, World Health Organization, 1211 Geneva 27, Switzerland).

Xerophthalmia

Sommer A. *Vitamin A deficiency and its consequences: a field guide to detection and control,* 3rd ed. Geneva, World Health Organization, 1995.

Vitamin A supplements: a guide to their use in the treatment and prevention of vitamin A deficiency and xerophthalmia. Geneva, World Health Organization, 1988.

The child, measles and the eye. Geneva, World Health Organization, 1993 (unpublished document WHO/EPI/TRAM/93.5, WHO/PBL/93.31; available on request from Programme for the Prevention of Blindness and Deafness, World Health Organization, 1211 Geneva 27, Switzerland).

Onchocerciasis

Strategies for ivermectin distribution through primary health care systems: report of the Meeting on Strategies for Ivermectin Distribution through Primary Health Care Systems, Geneva, 22–25 April 1991. Geneva, World Health Organization, 1991 (unpublished document WHO/PBL/91.24; available on request from Programme for the Prevention of Blindness and Deafness, World Health Organization, 1211 Geneva 27, Switzerland).

Onchocerciasis and its control. Report of a WHO Expert Committee on Onchocerciasis Control. Geneva, World Health Organization, 1995 (WHO Technical Report Series, No. 852).

Cataract

The provision of spectacles at low cost. Geneva, World Health Organization, 1987.
Management of cataract in primary health care services, 2nd ed. Geneva, World Health Organization, 1996.
Use of intraocular lenses in cataract surgery in developing countries: Memorandum from a WHO meeting. *Bulletin of the World Health Organization,* 1991, 69(6):657–666.

Ocular trauma

Thylefors B. Epidemiological patterns of ocular trauma. *Australia and New Zealand journal of ophthalmology,* 1992, 20(2):95–98.

Glaucoma

Thylefors B, Négrel A-D. The global impact of glaucoma. *Bulletin of the World Health Organization,* 1994, 72(3):323–326.

Diabetes mellitus

Prevention of diabetes mellitus. Report of a WHO Study Group. Geneva, World Health Organization, 1994 (WHO Technical Report Series, No. 844).

Childhood blindness

Prevention of childhood blindness. Geneva, World Health Organization, 1992.
Gilbert C et al. Childhood blindness: a new form for recording causes of visual loss in children. *Bulletin of the World Health Organization,* 1993, 71(5):485–489.
Conjunctivitis of the newborn: prevention and treatment at the primary health care level. Geneva, World Health Organization, 1986.
The multicenter trial of cryotherapy for retinopathy of prematurity. One-year outcome—structure and function. Cryotherapy for Retinopathy of Prematurity Cooperative Group. *Archives of ophthalmology,* 1990, 108:1408–1416.

General

WHO/PBL eye examination record. Geneva, World Health Organization, 1988 (unpublished document WHO/PBL/EER III/1988) and *Coding instructions;* (unpublished document PBL/88.1; available on request from Programme for the Prevention of Blindness and Deafness, World Health Organization, 1211 Geneva 27, Switzerland).
Formulation and management of national programmes for the prevention of blindness: suggested outlines. Geneva, World Health Organization, 1990 (unpublished document WHO/PBL/90.18; available on request from Programme for the Prevention of Blindness and Deafness, World Health Organization, 1211 Geneva 27, Switzerland).
The local small-scale preparation of eye drops. Geneva, World Health Organization, 1990 (unpublished document WHO/PBL/90.20; available on request from Programme

for the Prevention of Blindness and Deafness, World Health Organization, 1211 Geneva 27, Switzerland).

Thylefors B et al. Available data on blindness (update 1994). *Ophthalmic epidemiology*, 1995, 2:5–39.

Thylefors B et al. Global data on blindness. *Bulletin of the World Health Organization*, 1995, 73(1):115–121.

Management of low vision in children: report of a WHO consultation, Bangkok, 23–24 July 1992. Geneva, World Health Organization, 1993 (unpublished document WHO/PBL/93.27; available on request from Programme for the Prevention of Blindness and Deafness, World Health Organization, 1211 Geneva 27, Switzerland).